Praise for

LIFE AS WE KNEW IT

'It will be impossible not to find experiences and reactions that resonate in this remarkable compendium of our pandemic experience, but we are also challenged to learn through the eyes of others.

The authors astutely document political relationships, policy development, and at times deflection of responsibility, unafraid of sharing their views on key decisions and events, whilst remaining firmly focussed on the humanity of our response. The pain, loss, and scars of our experience are handled with care and compassion, and so too are the extraordinary stories of generosity and resilience.

In sharing the voices of our leaders, those at the pandemic frontline, and those most impacted, the authors draw together some of the lessons of the pandemic — the disparities in pandemic risk and response impacts, the shadow pandemic and mental health costs we are still learning about, and the forgotten children, key among them. A lack of nuance is another recurring theme — understandable, given the uncertainty at the start, but still pervasive years into the ordeal.

But most of all they remind us that everyone wanted Australia to do well — and we did. This is a story of success. It is our story.'

—Professor Catherine Bennett, epidemiology chair, Deakin University

LIFE AS WE KNEW IT

'Looking back, the Covid-19 pandemic seems like science fiction. So much has slipped from our memories. This account, which reads like a thriller, is a grim reminder that it can, or will, come around again. It reminds us of the successes and failures in Australia and elsewhere, and how luck can be as critical a factor as science. It could serve as a manual for how to respond in the future.'
—Jon Faine

'Closely reported, written with pace and acknowledging the personal, this is a must-read about Australia's unique experience of the pandemic.'
—Dr Norman Swan

LIFE AS WE KNEW IT

Aisha Dow is a multi-award-winning journalist and health editor based at *The Age* newspaper. She reported on the coronavirus pandemic for more than three years, through six lockdowns in Melbourne. Her investigations exposing the collapse of Victoria's triple-zero system, with her colleague Nick McKenzie, won a Walkley award. She previously worked on the city beat, uncovering a crisis of faulty, dangerous, and leaking buildings. She is a former Melbourne Press Club Young Journalist of the Year.

Melissa Cunningham is a multi-award-winning journalist based at *The Age* in Melbourne. She covered the coronavirus pandemic for more than three years as *The Age*'s health reporter through six lockdowns. Her news-breaking and investigative skills have been recognised by the Melbourne Press Club, which has awarded her two Quill awards for excellence in journalism. She was awarded for her extensive reporting on clergy and institutional sexual abuse in 2017, and won the best news story of the year in 2021 for a scoop exposing the failures of Victoria's hotel quarantine program. She has twice been a finalist in the Walkley awards. Cunningham loves telling people's stories, and values public interest journalism and its role in changing lives.

Aisha Dow and Melissa Cunningham

LIFE AS WE KNEW IT

the extraordinary story of Australia's pandemic

SCRIBE

Melbourne • London

Scribe Publications
18–20 Edward St, Brunswick, Victoria 3056, Australia
2 John St, Clerkenwell, London, WC1N 2ES, United Kingdom
3754 Pleasant Ave, Suite 100, Minneapolis, Minnesota 55409, USA

Published by Scribe 2023

Typeset in 11.25/15.75 pt Fairfield LT Std by the publishers

Printed and bound in Australia by Griffin Press

Scribe is committed to the sustainable use of natural resources and the use
of paper products made responsibly from those resources.

Scribe acknowledges Australia's First Nations peoples as the traditional
owners and custodians of this country, and we pay our respects to their
elders, past and present.

978 1 761380 03 7 (Australian edition)
978 1 761385 31 5 (ebook)

A catalogue record for this book is available from the National Library of
Australia.

scribepublications.com.au
scribepublications.co.uk
scribepublications.com

Contents

CHAPTER ONE

Something is happening in Wuhan

It was quite possibly the strangest moment of Professor Eddie Holmes' career. The eminent Australian scientist needed the services of a spy agency, but he wasn't sure how to contact one. 'Are they in the White Pages?' he joked, though he was worried too.

Exactly how he came to be in this predicament is a complicated tale. The short version is that Holmes and a couple of his international colleagues, all globally respected virologists, had suddenly become concerned that the new coronavirus discovered in the Chinese city of Wuhan showed signs of human influence. Was there an insert in the virus's genome? Had it come from a laboratory? This was why Holmes found himself asking around for the phone number of Australia's chief medical officer, Professor Brendan Murphy, expecting that he might be his best conduit to an Australian intelligence service. Holmes' associates in the United States and Britain promptly sought out their contacts at the CIA and MI5.

This is insane, Holmes thought, as he scoffed at someone's suggestion that he buy a burner phone. Soon he was in a teleconference discussing his and his colleague's concerns with an elite group of international scientists—among them, Anthony Fauci, a high-level adviser to US President Donald Trump. What happened in that meeting would become central to scores of conspiracy theories, and would be discussed and investigated for years to come.

If there was an Australian who had a front-row seat to the early twists and turns of the Covid-19 pandemic it was Holmes, even though, as time would tell, the concern that the contagion had signs of human intervention would recede in the minds of most of the top experts in disease spread. The focus would return to a Wuhan seafood market, where wild animals — racoon dogs and badgers, porcupines and hedgehogs — were stacked in narrow cages, and sold for food and fur. It was exactly the kind of place where a virus from a sick creature could spill over to humans, and the location near where most of the first cases of the nasty respiratory virus were clustered.

A few weeks earlier, on Sunday 5 January 2020. Holmes, a renowned global expert in the emergence of infectious diseases, was travelling with his wife and parents-in-law to a waterside café in Sydney's Pittwater when, just before 8.00 am, an email slipped into his inbox. 'Please call me immediately!!!' was the subject line. As he sat in the passenger seat of the family car, he dialled the eleven-digit international number listed in the email. At the end of the line was Chinese virologist Professor Yong-Zhen Zhang. His voice sounded anxious, but also tinged with excitement.

Moments before, Zhang and his team at the Shanghai Public Health Clinical Centre had finished mapping the genome of a virus that had appeared the month before in Wuhan, where it was causing a cluster of 'unusual pneumonia' cases in the bustling metropolis in China's east. A sample of the virus had been taken from the lung fluid of one of the workers at the market at the centre of the outbreak. Coughing, and with a high temperature, the man had arrived at hospital on 26 December 2019. The genome sequence revealed that the cause of the disease was alarmingly similar to SARS, another respiratory virus that had come out of China almost two decades earlier, killing more than 700 people before being eradicated in 2004 by intensive public health measures and a touch of luck.

'I remember the main thing we talked about was that "SARS was back." This was a huge thing,' said Holmes. 'I probably said,

"Oh, fuck."' As he disconnected the call and carefully put down his phone, his mother-in-law asked: 'What was that all about?' Even at this early stage, it was clear to Holmes that the disease in Wuhan was a new type of coronavirus and that it was spreading between humans. Coronaviruses are found in many different animal species, and include the common cold as well as far more serious infections such as SARS and MERS. 'This was not food poisoning from dodgy fish; case numbers were growing,' Holmes said. 'It was blindingly obvious that this was a human respiratory virus.'

At Holmes' urging, Zhang contacted China's National Health Commission the same day, advising the high-level department that the coronavirus his laboratory had sequenced that morning was similar to SARS, and that people needed to take precautions. The letter said that his unit at the Shanghai Public Health Clinical Centre had sequenced the entire genome of the virus that was causing febrile pneumonia of an unknown cause at the Huanan Seafood Market in Wuhan. The virus, which they had named Wuhan-Hu-1 Coronavirus, was 89.11 per cent homologous, meaning closely related, to the SARS coronavirus. 'Given that the virus is homologous to the coronavirus causing the SARS epidemic and should be transmitted via the respiratory tract, it is recommended that appropriate preventive and control measures be taken in public places as well as antiviral treatment be used in clinical care,' a translated version of the document said.

Was this a fleeting opportunity to circumvent the global pandemic? On this day, on 5 January, 59 cases of the disease had been officially detected, all within a single province in China. 'They had a chance to stop the pandemic,' Holmes insists. 'A series of mistakes were made,' he explained. 'The first mistake, though, was in Hubei province in Wuhan, where they should have clamped down really quickly, controlled and quarantined those cases, and they didn't do it.'

Several days before Zhang's letter was sent, a young Chinese doctor named Li Wenliang had also tried to sound the alarm about cases of a new coronavirus among patients in the Central Hospital of Wuhan. His efforts saw him reprimanded by local police, who issued a formal warning admonishing him for 'making false comments' that had 'severely disturbed the social order'. Tragically, the 34-year-old whistleblower died of Covid-19 in February the same year.

It would take until 20 January for Chinese officials to publicly confirm that they had evidence of human-to-human transmission, and longer before the residents of Wuhan were sent into the world's first Covid-19 lockdown. By the time the city was sealed off, at 10.00 am on 23 January, the disease had already made landfall in several other countries. Soon, hospitals as far away as the north of Italy were running out of intensive-care beds, forcing the rationing of care to the youngest and most likely to survive. In late March, the bodies began piling up in New York City. Refrigerated trucks rolled in to store the dead as the morgues were overrun, while authorities permitted cremations to run around the clock. In the United Kingdom, where the government had been slow to enforce a national lockdown, more than 1,000 people were dying each day by April 2020.

In those early weeks and months, even some of those working at the frontline of Australia's pandemic response believed the country would soon follow the United States and Europe into a catastrophe that was nearly impossible to circumvent. On 3 February, a hush fell over the boardroom at Scarborough House in Canberra when Australia's foremost public health officials were handed modelling from scientists at the nation's leading infectious diseases research centre, the Doherty Institute, and the University of Melbourne. *This is not controllable*, thought Professor Allen Cheng, as the infectious disease physician scanned a short document peppered with graphs. *This is going to come to Australia sometime, and it looks bad.*

In an interview with us three years later, Scott Morrison, who had been Australia's prime minister at the time, said those early months were marked by a deep uncertainty. 'I mean, no one knew what this thing was gonna do,' he said.

But then Australians met the challenge to 'flatten the curve' of the first-wave cases that arrived in the country in planeload after plane-load—they eradicated almost every infection that found its way into their cities and towns. Cases being detected fell from a national peak of almost 500 a day in late March 2020 to less than a dozen soon after, as domestic and international borders were closed. The public had been more compliant, and the strategy far more successful than predicted. Critically, the advice from Australia's world-class scientists and public health officials was heeded by political leaders in the nation's early response to the pandemic.

'There was no politics. We made these recommendations, and the government adopted them,' said epidemiologist and mathematical biologist Professor James McCaw, who worked as a high-level pandemic adviser to government. 'But it was massive. We were advising governments to fundamentally change society in a way that had never happened.'

Those two characteristics of the initial Australian response—the willingness of politicians to make extraordinary interventions on the back of expert advice, and a public spirit of collectivism over individualism—would be what would set Australia apart. A number of Australian scientists who were so influential in directing the nation's pandemic policies also played starring roles in the early global response to the spreading contagion.

Eddie Holmes, in the days after his initial phone call with Yong-Zhen Zhang, had been working with the Chinese virologist on a paper for the prestigious science journal *Nature*. In it, they were to describe the genome sequence of the new coronavirus. But there was something troubling Holmes. The detailed sequence, which would allow scientists to begin developing vaccines and tests for the new disease, still had not been publicly released. Holmes told us that Zhang was facing intense pressure from the Chinese authorities to keep things under wraps.

On the morning of Saturday 11 January, Holmes called Zhang as his plane was taxiing on a runway at Shanghai Hongqiao International Airport, en route to Beijing. Holmes could hear the final instructions of the cabin crew in Cantonese, telling people to buckle up. Holmes told him, 'We have to do it now.' Zhang asked the Australian scientist to give him a minute to think, and then he said, 'Okay.'

Holmes had the sequence for no more than an hour before he posted it online, uploading it at 12.05 pm Sydney time, on a website called virological.org. As he sat preparing the post in his small study with its brick walls and red-gum roof, he felt the full weight of the global responsibility. 'I remember I was trying to type, and I was so nervous I was making typos all over the place,' he said. 'I didn't even check the sequence once. I thought every minute I have it and it's not out there, is time lost. As soon as it was out there and I saw it online, I thought, *Oh, thank God.*'

Based on Zhang's sequence uploaded that afternoon from the Upper North Shore of Sydney, Moderna created its first mRNA Covid-19 vaccine, and it did it in less than two days. Zhang's self-less act was also credited with allowing scientists to develop the first rapid coronavirus tests. However, Holmes said the consequences for Zhang began immediately after he landed in Beijing a few hours later. He cannot say much more than this out of concern for his colleague. 'This is the great paradox of the whole thing. On the one hand, people are lauding the openness of the Chinese; on the other, the Chinese government clamped down, and they were absolutely furious.'

On the same day that Zhang's sequence was uploaded, China reported its first death from the pandemic—a 61-year-old man who had been a regular customer at the Wuhan seafood market.

As 2019 turned into 2020 in Australia, the coronavirus crisis arrived on the tail of another one. Bushfires of near-biblical propor-tions raged along the country, burning land equivalent to the size of the United Kingdom, and directly killing at least 33 people. Hundreds of millions of mammals, birds, reptiles, and invertebrates perished, almost certainly wiping out whole species of plants and animals.

On New Year's Eve, in the Victorian town of Mallacoota, residents and holidaymakers fled to the beach, and then in small boats out to sea, away from the gigantic, rapidly encroaching flames. Everything in the images from that time is bathed in apocalyptic red: the sky, the land, the haunted faces of the evacuees. In Melbourne, there were days when people couldn't see the end of their street because of the haze. The sky over Sydney turned orange.

When South Australia's chief public health officer, Nicola Spurrier, heard about a new virus in China around this time, her thoughts jumped to the size of Australia's stockpile of high-grade N95 masks, which were being stripped from hardware stores and chemists as the smoke spread. 'I remember thinking, *I hope that the national medical stockpile is pretty large, because I think we really have them for infectious diseases rather than bushfires,*' she said. 'Then, of course, we ended up with a pandemic.'

In Canberra, the smoke was so thick that Parliament House sunk into a grey pall. The nation's capital recorded the worst air quality in the world, and the public was urged to batten down and stay at home. Buried within the federal health department headquarters, the National Incident Room was busy with officials trying to manage the insidious health impacts of the fires.

Professor Paul Kelly, then Australia's acting chief medical officer, said he remembers being approached in the corridor by the coordinator of the emergency operations centre, Adam Lambert, who presented him with a new problem. 'I think something might be happening in Wuhan,' Lambert told him. Kelly said his immediate thoughts were, *Oh, not something else.* What was being described to him sounded very much like the original SARS. Kelly confessed that he didn't know where Wuhan, a city of 11 million people, was located. He had to google it. 'What I didn't know at that time, but found out quickly, was that there were direct flights from Wuhan to Australia several times a week.'

On 18 January, Queensland's chief health officer, Dr Jeannette Young, picked up her phone and called her husband, microbiologist Professor Graeme Nimmo, who was away for a weekend at Mooloolaba on the Sunshine Coast. 'Come home,' she told him. 'I need you.' Young had just left a teleconference with the nation's top public health officials in tears, already convinced that once the new coronavirus got into Australia, there would be no stopping it.

Her concern was telling; she was no rookie, but the nation's longest-serving chief health officer. The former emergency doctor had advised four premiers through the MERS outbreak in 2012, the swine flu pandemic in 2009, dengue outbreaks, and record-breaking influenza seasons.

Queensland's premier, Annastacia Palaszczuk, told us that when Young spoke, you listened. 'Dr Young was one of the most experienced health officers in the country. She's been there for a long time; she's seen a lot. She presented her advice to us, and said she believed that this pandemic was not going to be contained. What she says, you believe.'

At this time, Palaszczuk was also presented with modelling that predicted up to 30,000 deaths among Queenslanders, one in five people needing hospital treatment, and about a quarter of the population infected. Palaszczuk said it all felt so surreal. 'I thought, *Thirty thousand Queenslanders? They've all got families.*'

CHAPTER TWO

Landfall

The premier of Western Australia, Mark McGowan, had just spent a mild summer's day crabbing with his three children near Dawesville, a coastal suburb 85 kilometres south of Perth, when his phone lit up. It was Australia's prime minister, Scott Morrison. McGowan was covered in mud. His 11-year-old daughter, Amelia, was next to him, demanding tomato sauce for her pie. 'I kept telling her to be quiet and she wouldn't, so I had to keep talking to her while going into the bakery to buy some sauce as I spoke to the prime minister,' McGowan recalled. Morrison sounded tense as he briefed the premier. 'I'm going to have to shut down flights from China,' he said.

Many big and historic decisions would come in the days and months that followed, but this was the first. Morrison told us that it was on this day, Saturday 1 February 2020, that he began to really understand that the government would have to do things they would have never previously contemplated to get through what was beginning to look like a global pandemic. 'We knew in an open-trading economy like Australia, shutting the borders was a very big step to take,' he said. 'That was the very first large step to understanding this was going to hurt.'

The chain of events that culminated with a ban on foreigners who had recently been in China began with a midnight email from the director of epidemiology at the Doherty Institute, Professor Jodie McVernon, to Australia's chief medical officer, Brendan Murphy. McVernon had just seen a new paper, yet to be published. It estimated that about 76,000 people in Wuhan were already infected with the 'novel coronavirus', and that large overseas cities with close transport links to China would soon become virus epicentres, in the absence of substantial public health interventions. 'I didn't expect anyone to pick it [the email] up at that time,' McVernon recalled. 'But I didn't want to delay it, and I wanted it to be there when people woke up, saying this is important news.'

The next morning, Australia's health minister, Greg Hunt, was walking laps of the oval in the rain at his son's cricket match at Balnarring, a tiny town on Victoria's Mornington Peninsula, when he received a call from Murphy. The chief medical officer was suggesting to Hunt something that, less than two weeks earlier, would have been inconceivable. 'On the 19th of January, the idea that we would suddenly be closing the border with China for some still-to-be determined reason was virtually unimaginable,' Hunt said. 'That decision is arguably the most important peacetime decision Australia has made in the last 50 years … it set the tone for everything.'

But before Hunt had a chance to call the prime minister, his phone started buzzing. Morrison, who was sorting through morning reports at his official Sydney residence, Kirribilli House, had also been thinking about border controls. The prime minister and the health minister had been friends for years, and, in the words of Morrison, 'could largely read each other's mind and finish each other's sentences'. Morrison, Hunt, and Murphy joined a three-way call later that morning, and the chief medical officer repeated his belief that Australia needed to act immediately in the face of the 'clear and present' danger that the new coronavirus posed to the country. Meetings of the National Security Committee and Australian Health Protection Principal Committee were hastily called. Australian

Border Force commissioner Michael Outram advised Hunt that it would be able to close Australia's border to China within 12 hours. China was notified of the decision.

Morrison called the state premiers and the New Zealand prime minister, Jacinda Ardern, to give them a heads-up. By 5.00 pm, the prime minister and the foreign affairs minister, Marise Payne, were stepping out to announce that foreign nationals in mainland China would not be allowed to enter Australia for 14 days after leaving China, effective immediately. Australian citizens and permanent residents arriving from China would have to isolate at home for 14 days.

Murphy, a nephrologist who emerged from relative obscurity to become a popular and reassuring public figure during the early months of the pandemic in Australia, said he was struck by the heady pace of the decision-making at the time. 'The idea that I would wake up on a Saturday morning at nine o'clock, and would start a process that would lead to borders being closed to China at nine o'clock that night, I mean those sort of things are sort of unimaginable in most lives.'

On 21 January, Murphy had declared the new coronavirus a disease of pandemic potential under Australia's Biosecurity Act, triggering a string of pandemic-preparedness measures, including daily meetings of the states' chief health officers. This was more than a week ahead of the World Health Organisation's move to declare the outbreak of the novel coronavirus as a 'public health emergency of international concern'.

'Oh yeah, they'll sort it out,' was Jodie McVernon's casual assessment the first time she was told about what would later become known as Covid-19. Her sister, a lawyer, had mentioned she had heard of a strange new pneumonia in China, at a time when the accounts of the outbreak were still buried in newspapers' back pages. 'I was so wrong,' said the mathematical modeller of infectious diseases, with a wry smile. 'So [my sister] likes to point out that she knew about it before me.'

McVernon and her colleague at the Doherty Institute, Professor James McCaw, were Australia's leading experts in pandemic prepared-ness, having spent the previous 15 years working on complex disease modelling and helping to develop Australia's pandemic plan. McCaw, a professor of mathematical biology at the University of Melbourne, had spent his career studying infectious diseases. His frank, calm advice would be sought many times by governments, health offi-cials, and journalists. McVernon was one Australia's most influential epidemiologists. Although she was often sought for her views, she remained a reluctant public figure.

On 17 January, the pair were among the first to see and be rocked by influential papers from researchers at the Imperial College London. Along with other leading infectious disease modellers from across the globe, they joined an evening conference call arranged by the World Health Organisation, where they listened to a presenta-tion from Professor Neil Ferguson, a prominent expert in the mathe-matical modelling of infectious diseases. Forty-one cases of the new coronavirus had been officially detected in Wuhan, in addition to two cases in Thailand and one in Japan — travellers who had recently been in the Chinese city. However, according to the 17 January report from Ferguson and his team, the real number of cases was higher, dramatically so. They put the likely figure as being closer to 1,723, and possibly much more.

As the Chinese New Year approached, when millions would travel across China and the globe to see their families, a list was published in an academic paper of the top 20 destinations for travellers from Wuhan. Sydney and Melbourne were among them. If McVernon's initial reaction was a little blasé, it would be swiftly replaced with an uncomfortable certainty that the new virus that was spreading around the world was most certainly going to be bad. The question that remained was precisely how bad.

For weeks in January, one of Melbourne's most-experienced infectious disease physicians, Professor Rhonda Stuart, had been on high alert. It was late on Friday 24 January when she got the call she had been waiting for. A man from China in his 50s who had recently spent two weeks in the virus's epicentre, Wuhan, who had been visiting his daughter in Melbourne, was in the hospital's emergency department. He had arrived at the Monash Medical Centre, in the city's south-east, with a high fever and a dry cough, and had quickly been taken to an isolation room. Stuart remembers calling the health service's chief executive, Professor Andrew Stripp, to tell him about the potential case, before racing down to the emergency department to assist the team caring for him. 'When I got that call on that day, there was no doubt in my mind that this was it,' Stuart said.

A zip-lock bag with a sample from the man's nose and throat was ferried across town into the brown office tower housing the Doherty Institute. Soon after, a pair of senior virologists, Dr Julian Druce and Dr Mike Catton, were working on a rather mundane task, pulling together staff rosters, when two duty scientists suddenly appeared at the door of their meeting room. They had news. The test result was back. It showed that SARS-CoV-2 had been detected in Australia for the first time. Druce and Catton ran a second test, just to be sure, amplifying a large chunk of the virus's genetic code. It revealed a match for the genomic sequence that Professor Eddie Holmes had uploaded almost two weeks earlier.

While most diagnostic labs around the world use genetic sequencing to test for viruses, the Doherty Institute was one of the few to keep extensive cell lines, which allowed the scientists to do something else that would be critical to understanding and preparing for the virus: growing it. No other lab had yet been able to achieve this feat outside China, and the Chinese were yet to share the virus with the rest of the world.

Julian Druce, the head of the Doherty's virus-identification laboratory, had a reputation for having 'green fingers' when it came to growing tricky viruses. He placed material from the infected man in a small plastic flask filled with a layer of monkey cells, and then he and his team waited. It was Sunday afternoon when Druce ventured back into the laboratory, wearing his casual weekend uniform of jeans and a T-shirt, and peered into a microscope. It looked like something was happening. He set up a video on the microscope so he could watch from home. More wiggling black dots were appearing in the images, taken every 15 minutes. These were the tantalising early signs that the virus was replicating.

When the virologists looked over the final test the following Tuesday morning, a camera crew from the ABC just happened to be at the laboratory filming for another story. 'We've got it!' said Catton in the vision captured by the news crew, as the pair gathered around the test readout showing that the virus was 1,000 times stronger than when it was first measured. 'Fantastic!' The breakthrough was described as a 'game changer'. It meant that samples of the virus grown in the Melbourne laboratory could be used to check the accuracy of tests being developed, and could help in the development of vaccines.

Test tubes of pink liquid containing the virus were packed into boxes of dry ice at the Doherty building in Melbourne, and flown to dozens of labs across Australia and the globe. The World Health Organisation assisted in the process, while Australia's Defence Export Controls Branch helped with screening labs receiving the live agent.

Aided by the virus samples, Australia would quite quickly establish a robust Covid-19 testing system. In contrast, early testing failures in the United States resulted in what would later be described as a 'lost month' that rendered the country blind to the scale of the catastrophe ahead.

Australia's first case of Covid-19 was publicly announced on the morning of Saturday 25 January. Later that day, three other men were also confirmed to be infected with the virus in New South Wales. Two had flown in from Wuhan, and the third from another Chinese city, Shenzhen. A televised press conference was called, and prime minister Scott Morrison urged Australians not to panic, telling viewers that the federal government was 'taking this issue incredibly seriously' and had 'activated the necessary precautions and procedures'.

It was around the same time that the notion that Covid-19 had escaped from a Chinese laboratory began to be seriously considered by the who's who of infectious diseases. Eddie Holmes was making his way home from a virology conference in Switzerland when he received an email from British infectious disease researcher Sir Jeremy Farrar. It said, 'There is talk in the US that this virus might be out of a lab.'

In late January 2020, the closest known relation to the new coronavirus, SARS-CoV-2, was a type of coronavirus called RaTG13, found in horseshoe bats from Yunnan province in south-western China. In a twist of sorts that would fuel the laboratory-escape theory for years to come, RaTG13 was being studied at the Wuhan Institute of Virology, about 30 kilometres from the Wuhan seafood market. However, RaTG13 is not the direct ancestor of Covid-19, and scientists believe it's so distantly related that it couldn't be engineered to create Covid-19. Closer relatives to Covid-19 have since been found, although still no direct ancestor, leaving a remaining mystery about the pandemic's origin.

Holmes said he was not overly concerned by the loose link between RaTG13 and the new coronavirus. But the next day, he got a Zoom call from Professor Kristian Andersen, a Danish evolutionary biologist based in California, who thought he could see what looked like a human-made insert in the genome.

'Then it went from zero to 100 really quickly,' Holmes recalled. 'Immediately, I called Jeremy [Farrar] back and said, "Look, we've got a problem — this could be engineered." He said, "You need to talk to your local intelligence services, I'll talk to M15, Kristian can call the CIA."' Holmes got in touch with a colleague at the University of Sydney, Australian infectious disease physician Tania Sorrell, who was able to arrange for Australia's chief medical officer, Professor Murphy, to call him. 'I think he said "Geez" a lot,' said Holmes of that short conversation with Murphy. Holmes said he was then called by

Nick Warner, the head of Australia's Office of National Intelligence, and he spoke to him and a number of other people in the intelligence agency several times. 'It was like spy stuff, very cloak-and-dagger. I don't go around talking to intelligence services on a daily basis. It's not part of my work, so the whole thing was just surreal.'

Holmes helped to quickly convene the now-infamous teleconference with some of the biggest global names in infectious diseases and virology on Saturday 2 February. They included Anthony Fauci, the director of the US National Institute of Allergy and Infectious Diseases; Francis Collins, the director of the US National Institutes of Health; and virologists Christian Drosten and Marion Koopmans. The audio hook-up was at 6.00 am Sydney time. Holmes hadn't slept well the night before because he was so worried.

'Kristian spoke first; he presented some data. I spoke second. Then we had a robust discussion about it.' The scientists' overwhelming concern related to a tiny piece of genetic code in the virus called a furin cleavage site.

Furin cleavage sites regularly appear in viruses, and can allow them to better infect human cells. What initially seemed so strange about the site in SARS-CoV-2 was that it was not found in any of its closest relatives, the coronaviruses found in bats. Worryingly, it was also flanked by 'molecular scissor cuts', known as restriction enzyme sites, which scientists commonly use to edit gene sequences. To Holmes and Andersen, this appeared like the signature of human engineering. 'The furin cleavage site looked like it had been cut-and-pasted in,' Holmes said.

However, Holmes said that when the scientists looked more carefully, they discovered that the restriction enzyme sites were actually occurring naturally over the SARS-CoV-2 genome. 'So that what we observed meant nothing.'

During the teleconference, which lasted about an hour, Holmes said that Dutch virologist Ron Fouchier, Christian Drosten, and Marion Koopmans argued to varying degrees against the idea that the new coronavirus had been engineered, 'and they made very good points'. He described it as a 'nerdy science discussion'.

'My own view changed very quickly. So on 31 January and 1 February, I was probably very worried. And by 4 or 5 February I wasn't worried.'

Soon after that meeting, the sequence of a coronavirus from a pangolin, a kind of scaly anteater, became available, showing a remarkable similarity to Covid-19 in some genes. 'This really made SARS-CoV-2 look like just another natural virus,' Holmes noted.

But conspiracy theorists and elements of the media, particularly in the US, later latched onto this swift shift in opinion as a sign of something nefarious. 'What happened at the February 1 teleconference to make the virologists change their minds so radically?' wrote journalist Nicholas Wade in 2022. One of the ideas that has gained considerable traction is that the mild-mannered Fauci, alongside another of America's most respected scientists, Francis Collins, bullied scientists, including Holmes, to reverse their position because the US had been funding the Wuhan lab to do controversial experiments. Although a small amount of US money had gone to a project examining the risk of coronavirus emerging from wildlife, whether any US money was used to make viruses more dangerous in order to study them is disputed.

Holmes, one of about a dozen people at the meeting, said it was 'complete bullshit' that he was pressured to change his view. 'Fauci and Collins didn't say much at all,' he said. 'All they wanted to know was, "What does the science say?" It was as simple as that. They didn't guide us.'

Fauci told news outlet *US Today* in 2021: 'I always had an open mind … even though I felt then, and still do, the most likely origin was in an animal host.'

While outsiders see conspiracies, scientists will explain it is not unusual that experts will disagree, test theories, or change their minds—even more so at a time when the knowledge of the virus was in its infancy. Still, the lab-leak theory has gained so much attention, promoted by US president Donald Trump, who claimed his administration had evidence the virus had originated from the lab, that it has become mainstream in America. In December 2022, Twitter's billionaire owner, Elon Musk, tweeted that Fauci should be prosecuted for lying to Congress and funding dangerous research 'that killed millions of people'.

For many, Holmes is an evil player in a conspiracy to cover up one of the world's greatest scandals. He said he has learnt not to let it bother him, but there's no doubt that the constant accusations and noise are consuming, distracting, and often just plain wild. For a period, Kristian Andersen in California had armed security guarding him around the clock. Virologist Robert Garry, also part of the February teleconference call, had rocks thrown at his New Orleans home.

Republican politicians in the US were investigating the origins of the virus in 2023. Holmes said that he expected to get the call to testify, and would probably attend, even though as an Australian he wouldn't be legally required to, 'because I don't mind having a row'. They want this to be Watergate, but Fauci is not Nixon, and [all the other scientists on the teleconference] are not all the president's men,' he said.

As the pandemic progressed, Holmes became a leading researcher on the origins of Covid-19 and a prominent proponent of the case that the virus had emerged from an animal, most likely at the Huanan Seafood Wholesale Market. 'The lab-leak theory rests on an unfortunate coincidence: that SARS-CoV-2 emerged in a city with a laboratory that works on bat coronaviruses,' the scientist wrote in an opinion piece in 2022. 'Some of these bat coronaviruses are closely related to SARS-CoV-2. But not close enough to be direct ancestors.'

Because the animal that passed Covid-19 on to humans has not been identified, it's not possible to rule out the lab-leak theory entirely, but nor is there evidence that SARS-CoV-2 was kept in the Wuhan lab, let alone that it escaped or was released from there. One of the pieces of evidence in favour of the natural-origins theory is that two distinct lineages of Covid-19 were discovered in Wuhan early in the pandemic, suggesting that the virus had been circulating in animals for long enough to split into multiple variants before being picked up by humans.

Lab-leak advocates have tried to dismiss the clustering of the early cases around the Huanan Seafood Wholesale Market, arguing it is the perfect place the virus would spread from an infected laboratory worker, for example. But a 2022 study published in the prestigious *Science* journal by Holmes, Andersen, and others found that the market was not a popular location in the city at all. It wasn't even a very popular market. There were at least 70 other markets that received more social media check-ins. Holmes described it as like 'going to Coles in Bendigo on a wet Wednesday afternoon'.

The Age's national science reporter, Liam Mannix, said, 'Once you come in with the mindset *China has done the wrong thing*, you can go to an awful lot of effort trying to force the evidence to suit your perspective. And I think that's really what's happened here.' Mannix argued that putting undeserved focus on the lab-leak theory is especially unhelpful when it distracts governments and the world at large from doing the things that might help prevent the next pandemic. 'The natural-origin theory of Covid-19 says that the pandemic was both random chance, but also our fault: the climate crisis, deforestation, animal trafficking, mega-cities, air travel, and intensive agriculture have all been dramatically increasing our risks of a pandemic,' he said. 'Fixing that will be hard, and necessitates uncomfortable conversations about how we live now.'

Worryingly, China, which has a history of seeding animal-based pandemics and an active live wildlife trade, has also responded to the unsupported hypothesis about its nefarious role in the pandemic by offering its own conspiracy theories, including the idea that American soldiers began the pandemic in Wuhan. None of this helps the underlying issues and causes to be addressed.

So what did Holmes think happened? He said that a coronavirus probably passed from a horseshoe bat and onto an intermediary animal, such as a raccoon dog or a civet, before the sickness moved onto its first human hosts at the Wuhan market, and then on and on. This is how most other pandemics have occurred: a virus spills from animals to humans. The original SARS has been linked to civets, a possum-like wild mammal, also eaten in China.

The market-origin theory was further bolstered when, in 2023, Chinese scientists uploaded raw data to an online international repository. It revealed there was genetic material belonging to many wild animals in Covid-positive swabs taken from the Huanan market around January 2020, including large amounts that were a match for the raccoon dog, a fox-like animal known to be susceptible to coronavirus.

It was still not definitive proof that Covid-19 had come from wild animals at the market. However, Stephen Goldstein, a virologist at the University of Utah who was involved in analysing the data, explained: 'If you were to go and do environmental sampling in the aftermath of a zoonotic spillover event … this is basically exactly what you would expect to find.'

The Huanan Seafood Market has almost always been the prime suspect. In January 2020, it was shuttered. Orange barricades were placed across its entry point, and masked security guards patrolled its perimeters. The surrounding mega-city was desolate. Those who remained in Wuhan said the atmosphere resembled a scene from a Hollywood disaster movie. Locals, tourists, and expats barricaded themselves indoors. Every morning, expat Melbourne horse trainer Rui Severino had his temperature taken by a guard posted outside his building. 'Anyone who has a temperature higher than normal, you get reported and you get taken away,' he said in late January 2020. 'Everyone is extremely fearful, and that is why we must follow the measures enforced by the Chinese government very strictly.'

On 3 February, 200 Australian citizens and 43 permanent residents were flown from Wuhan on a chartered Qantas evacuation flight, navigating the roadblocks through the city with passes arranged by Australian officials. Qantas would embark on a further two rescue flights in the weeks that followed. The first group were taken to an air force base on the north-west desert coast of Western Australia, where they were to be transferred to several smaller planes bound for Christmas Island in the Indian Ocean. The island's immigration detention centre had been repurposed as a temporary quarantine station.

Waiting in the dark at the Learmonth air force base to receive them was the country's chief nursing and midwifery officer, Professor Alison McMillan, and a small group of staff from the Australian Medical Assistance Team. It was about 27 degrees when the Qantas Boeing 747 landed. The relieved passengers, eager to disembark, were still in their winter puffer jackets and jumpers. McMillan recalls the distress of a woman travelling with her three children under six, who had been forced to leave her husband, barred from joining the flight because he had a temperature. 'She had no idea what had happened to her husband ... [we were] trying to support and help with the little ones,' she said. 'We took the vulnerable out first—the families, the kids, the elderly.'

It was during this same week that the Doherty Institute modellers were approached by Brendan Murphy and asked to provide some scenarios describing how the new virus might spread in Australia. They did this by using very early estimates of its reproduction number—essentially a measure of how contagious it was—and an assumption that it would spread about as quickly as the original SARS virus. They already knew that people would be infectious for around a week. Using these three measurements, they drew epidemic curves showing how many people would become infected if Australia was to simply let the virus spread.

Ever since then, some people have repeatedly misrepresented such modelling as failed 'predictions'. In fact, the 'if' in the worst-case scenario that the modellers presented was hypothetical. As modeller James McCaw is keen to point out, the government was never going to let a potentially fatal disease spread completely unchecked. Still, the modelling did come back with a worrying conclusion. 'We looked at a few different severity levels. What if the virus is really dangerous? What happens if it's mildly dangerous? All of them said that this is going to be very bad. And we have to do something,' McCaw said.

A few weeks earlier, McCaw and McVernon were asked to join the Australian Health Protection Principal Committee, at a time when the group, known often by its acronym AHPPC, was almost as little known as its members. Chaired by Australia's chief medical officer, it was largely made up of the state's chief public health officers: New South Wales' Kerry Chant; Victoria's Brett Sutton; Queensland's Jeannette Young; South Australia's Nicola Spurrier; Western Australia's Andy Robertson; and Tasmania's Mark Veitch. The Northern Territory was represented by Hugh Heggie, and the Australian Capital Territory by Kerryn Coleman.

None of these people had any real public profile to speak of before the pandemic. In fact, they were so far from the spotlight that one of the state's chief health officers joked that although they had been in the job for many years, it was the first time a health minister had known their name. Previously, the public profile of the bureaucrats had generally been confined to alerts on less-momentous public health concerns: new measles cases, a flesh-eating ulcer epidemic, syphilis cases on the rise, and a hepatitis A outbreak. Whether they liked it or not, Australia's chief health officers would be pushed out of the shadows, often fronting near-daily live press conferences alongside their premier, subject to an extreme level of scrutiny as they made enormous decisions impacting lives and livelihoods.

James McCaw said that the period in late January and early February 2020 was very confronting, personally and professionally, because he was acutely aware that he was now part of a team of experts and officials who would be instrumental in shaping what was written in the history books. 'I knew we were faced with something that was going to be global news for a long time,' he said. 'AHPPC was going to be very influential. And if it did its job, it could save hundreds to tens of thousands of lives in Australia. If it didn't do its job, maybe it wouldn't.'

There was a period when, perhaps, Australia's top health officials thought there was nothing that they *could* do. McCaw recalls when the AHPPC was first presented with coronavirus modelling in early February, it showed the scale of the potential catastrophe, but also something else: if people made relatively small changes to their behaviour, such as meeting 25 per cent fewer people, there would be a huge reduction in the number of people infected and killed.

According to McCaw's account, New South Wales' chief health officer, Dr Kerry Chant, looked at these projections and said: 'Oh we can do something about this.' McCaw replied: 'Yes, we can.' The epidemiologist said it was a powerful moment, because he felt some of the chief health officers might have thought that there was nothing they could do, that 'it was just going to wash over us, and we would just be picking up the pieces. And Kerry realised that maybe we could do something'.

In early March, there was another galvanising moment. One of Australia's well-known public health experts, Dr Craig Dalton, had just read an interview with Dr Bruce Aylward, the scientist who had led the World Health Organisation delegation to China to investigate the Covid-19 outbreak the month before. Before he had read the piece, he said he shared the same view of most of Australia's public health experts: the country had little choice but to let the virus run its course. On 5 March, Dalton sent out an email to dozens of other leading public health officials, summarising what he had learnt and setting out his subsequent change of view. He told them it was dangerous and incorrect to assume that Australia had a superior medical capacity to China, and that the Chinese had in fact been able to save more lives than might have been expected in Western medical facilities. 'If we don't go as hard as China, we could have a worse outcome than Wuhan,' he wrote.

Dalton also began lobbying the federal health department to invite Bruce Aylward to give an address to Australian public health officials. When that didn't work, he quickly created a new 'front organisation' with a sufficiently official-sounding name: the Australian Health

Protection Officers Association, and made the approach himself. On a Friday evening, 6 March, the association held its inaugural meeting. About 70 public health practitioners joined a webinar with Aylward. The sandy-haired scientist barely paused for breath as he laid down what he knew. From his low-key office, a busy in-tray behind him, Aylward repeated his message: the new coronavirus was not the flu. 'The big, big message is you really want to try to contain this,' he told the Australian officials. 'A substantial proportion of your population is at high risk for mortality with this disease.'

Among those who tuned into the webinar was South Australia's chief public health officer, Professor Nicola Spurrier. She said the presentation was excellent, but also frightening. As Aylward talked, she took reams of notes, underlining key points for emphasis. 'He was saying, *Take this seriously. China has a very sophisticated health-care system. They are really putting every effort into controlling this, because it's very, very serious.*' Before the video conference, Spurrier said the thinking was that the new coronavirus would be like a 'something like a bad flu', but Aylward's testimony shook this view, and his message stuck with her: if it was possible to stop the virus coming to Australia before its population was protected by vaccines, they should grab that opportunity.

The situation in Italy, where the coronavirus death toll had surpassed 100, was alarming, but the worst was still around the corner, as many people would get progressively sicker from the disease over weeks. 'To die, it can take quite a long time,' Aylward noted. At the end of the presentation, Dalton thanked Aylward for his time, telling him that he suspected his webinar might have saved tens of thousands of Australian lives.

Later, Dalton told us he thought the presentation was critical to influencing Australia's response because, beforehand, some of the chief health officers had believed they couldn't stop the virus taking hold. 'Bruce gave such an inspirational presentation and convinced us that it was possible, that you had to believe it was possible, and I think that changed a lot of people's attitudes that this could be done.'

After he finished his address, Aylward said that when he had been asked to do the talk, he'd considered a debt of sorts he'd owed the country. 'Australia was very, very good to me when I had metastatic melanoma 15 years ago, and you guys took care of me. I'm still alive. I owe you guys a lot. You never forget these things.'

Certainly, the presentation was a lightbulb moment for Spurrier in South Australia about the seriousness of the threat posed by coronavirus. 'I thought, *Thank goodness I've taken all these notes*, and then I went running around, showing everybody in the department, [saying] "This is serious."'

CHAPTER THREE

Down in the dumps

Tucked away on the edge of the South Australian country town of Millicent, amid sundried farmland, is a toilet paper factory. From the outside, it looks fairly unremarkable: a collection of white warehouses behind a chain-wire fence. Before the pandemic, even some locals didn't realise it had been there for 60 years, or that the manufacturing facility produced enough toilet paper to supply roughly one-third of Australia's population. All of this made the appearance of a small fleet of media trucks that rolled into town from Adelaide in the early days of March 2020 all the more remarkable. Suddenly, national television breakfast show *Sunrise* was crossing live to a warehouses piled near to the ceiling with Kleenex toilet paper.

'Now to the topic everyone is talking about this morning,' began co-host David Koch, as he introduced the segment from the show's studio on Martin Place in Sydney. 'Supermarkets across Australia have been running out of dunny paper before it even hits the shelves. There have been extraordinary scenes right around the country—swarms of people racing to grab as many rolls as they can, amid fears about coronavirus.'

Co-presenter Samantha Armytage threw live to a distribution

centre, where forklifts were bustling in the background, while Kleenex senior marketing manager Gabbi Davidson reassured the nation that they were not at risk of running out of toilet paper. There was some semi-serious talk about supply chains, raw materials, and police escorts before the conversation turned towards folding versus scrunching one's toilet paper.

'What are you, Gabbi? Are you a folder or a scruncher?' asked Koch.

'I said she didn't have to answer that!' protested Armytage, despite having brought up the topic to begin with.

'I'm a scruncher,' replied Davidson. 'And I'm proud of it, it's fine.'

By 3 March, the panic buying was so widespread that prime minister Scott Morrison made a rare call to officials at the country's leading supermarkets, Coles and Woolworths, to discuss the problem.

There were several ugly incidents involving shoppers. Footage of three women in a violent tussle at the Chullora Woolworths in Sydney over a jumbo pack of Quilton toilet paper went viral on social media, and made global news. A mother and her adult daughter reportedly gave chase to another shopper who had, allegedly, snatched one of eight very large packets of toilet paper out of their trolley. The pair managed to retrieve the packet and, in the aftermath of the scuffle, could be seen guarding their loot. In the video of that incident, they place their hands defensively over their trolley, filled beyond the brim with loo paper. A supermarket worker scolds them. 'Look what you're doing, you're fighting over tissues,' she says. Another similar video taken in a Coles supermarket in early March showed the aftermath of a fight between two women. One has grey hair and glasses, and can be seen slapping her hand towards the face of a much younger woman, who already has a trolley full of paper in assorted brands. Bystanders are appalled. 'It's toilet paper!' says a young man, who comes in to break up the pair. The older woman retreats, triumphantly, with the disputed packet.

Supermarkets soon implemented buying limits for toilet paper. By the time the *Sunrise* segment went to air, Woolworths had rationed buyers to four packets per customer, and the Kimberly-Clark plant in Millicent was having to put in place unprecedented measures, too. Workers at the mill were accustomed to ramping up production of tissues during what they dubbed the 'sneazon season'—the traditional cold and flu period. Demand for toilet paper had always stayed pretty steady throughout the year, until now. Mill manager Adam Carpenter said he had worked for Kimberly-Clark for over 20 years, 'and I can clearly say it was the first time I'd experienced anything as dramatic'. Even the towns of Millicent and nearby Mount Gambier, where many of the 400 staff lived, were not immune to the toilet paper shortages, as the local supermarkets were supplied by the same distribution channels as the rest of the country. Carpenter said that they gave workers enough toilet paper to see them through the shortage period.

'The average consumption is a roll per person, per week,' he explained. 'So as long as we were providing enough to cover a family of four or five, they would be sure to have enough.' For about eight weeks in March and April 2020, the toilet paper factory was well and truly on the map. It was hard to miss the 50 semi-trailers parked along each side of the road on the grassy or gravel verges at the entry of the mill. Over that period, Carpenter said they would have expected to dispatch 1.7 million cases of product. Instead, more than 2.4 million were packed into the waiting trucks. Toilet paper production increased to 1.2 million rolls a day, a rate Carpenter said was sustained for years after the initial period of panic buying, as global shipping problems reduced competitor's imports.

Longtime Woolworths shelf-stacker Jake Vassallo recalled that the early 2020 rush on supermarkets persisted for months, and the volume of the daily load of groceries coming into his store at Epping in Melbourne's outer-northern suburbs was consistently as large as what they would usually see during the Christmas week. He said that, for a time, the supermarket's opening hours were cut because people were buying so many groceries the store couldn't keep up and needed more time for staff to focus on restocking shelves. It was exhausting work, compounded by the behaviour of some shoppers, who would yell and swear at workers because of the long waits to be served. 'It was a scary time for the staff, too. We were all worried about catching coronavirus, because we didn't know what it was, and on top of that we had customers abusing us because we just couldn't serve them quick enough,' Vassallo remembered. He worked along-side emergency workers brought in to fill the roster, among them grounded airline staff from Australia's national carrier, Qantas. An out-of-work pilot filled online orders.

One evening at the supermarket, Vassallo witnessed a verbal altercation break out between two customers. A middle-aged man had grabbed a packet of toilet paper directly from the trolley of an older woman. The man yelled that the woman 'had enough' of them. Vassallo had worked at Woolworths for more than a decade, since he was a teenager, and said security guards had never been needed until now. To avoid chaos in the toilet paper aisle, Vassallo said staff at the Epping store had to keep pallets of it inside the storeroom, and hand it out to customers queuing at the storeroom door.

It was around this time, as tensions boiled over, that Matt Williams, the editor of the Northern Territory's daily tabloid news-paper, the NT News, received an email from a colleague in Adelaide suggesting that he print a couple of blank pages of newspaper as mock 'toilet paper'. His colleague worked at The Advertiser, South Australia's more staid daily tabloid, where such a gimmick may not have been so well received. But he figured it could be just the thing for the NT News, which has never been averse to a toilet joke, and has somewhat of a global reputation for not taking itself too seriously. Notable past headlines have included 'The Poogitive', about a bikie who had landed face-first in a pile of manure while fleeing police, and a front-page 'Expoosive' with the story of a 'crap night out' of taxi driver whose customer had offloaded 'a massive steamer during the drive home'.

Williams said he took his colleague's advice, then went a step further, calling edition control and asking them to increase the size of the next day's paper, not by two pages, but by eight pages in the middle, which would be dedicated to sheets of 'toilet paper' adorned with the NT News logo. The banner on the front page of the newspaper on 5 March declared: 'Run out of loo paper? The NT News cares. That's why we've printed an EIGHT-PAGE special liftout inside, complete with handy cut lines, for you to use in an emergency. Get your limited edition one-ply toilet newspaper sheets.'

Williams doesn't know if anyone used the 'toilet paper', and that wasn't the intention. But the move did create plenty of headlines. 'I remember at the time, everyone was a bit down in the dumps about the whole thing,' Williams recalled. 'So we sort of saw it as a thing where we could lift people's spirits a bit and give them a bit of a laugh. That appeared to do the trick.'

For a time, it seemed that the real crisis was being obscured by a trivial, manufactured one. As Australians were being schooled on the importance of social distancing, they jostled among crowds of shoppers for a packet of toilet paper they didn't really need, and impatiently tapped harried supermarket workers on the shoulder. When recalling this time in the pandemic, many Australians will tell you that they are struck by their naivety in those days and weeks. This wouldn't last much longer.

CHAPTER FOUR

Australia wakes up

As the plane to Sydney streaked across Australia's red centre, the Northern Territory's chief minister, Michael Gunner, wondered to himself, *Is this really a wise thing to do?* The 45-year-old Labor leader was recovering from a very recent heart attack that had required surgery. His first baby was on the way. Life was moving quickly, and the more he heard about coronavirus from the territory's medical team, the more concerned he became.

The day he left Darwin, on 12 March 2020, a $17.6 billion economic-support package was announced by prime minister Scott Morrison and treasurer Josh Frydenberg, although more would soon be needed. *Do we really want every head of government in one spot at the one time?* thought Gunner. *Surely they'll cancel, right?* Yet, not long after, Gunner was passing through the black iron gates at Kirribilli House, prime minister Scott Morrison's official residence in Sydney. Also meeting Morrison for dinner and drinks were the seven other state and territory leaders, before what would be the last meeting of the Council of Australian Governments (COAG), the traditional forum for negotiations between the states and the federal government.

As the other leaders dispersed to their homes and hotels later that evening, Victorian premier Daniel Andrews stayed back to catch a moment with the prime minister. The powerful leaders from opposite sides of Australia's political divide sat on the back porch of the grand residence, each gripping a glass of single-malt Tasmanian whisky. Andrews was getting text messages about the Australian Grand Prix, due to begin in Melbourne the next day, amid raging speculation over whether it was safe to proceed. The pair agreed that night that Morrison would travel down to Melbourne, and they would appear together on Eddie McGuire's radio show 'to try to calm people about everything and show a bit of united front'. But things were changing fast, and the radio appearance never eventuated.

Seven hundred kilometres away in Melbourne, a senior infectious disease physician at the Alfred Hospital, Professor Allen Cheng, picked up the phone and dialled Victoria's chief health officer, Brett Sutton. Not long before, the hospital had received a test swab belonging to a McLaren mechanic, a member of one of the Formula One teams due to compete the following day at the Grand Prix. It had come back positive for coronavirus, Cheng told Sutton. Victoria's top public health official and his team now had an unenviable call to make: let the Grand Prix proceed and risk a catastrophic super-spreading event, or call it off with just hours to go, wasting many millions of dollars and disappointing hundreds of thousands of fans.

'He doesn't give much away, Brett, with what he is thinking, but you could see that the wheels were turning,' recalled Cheng. At 1.00 am, Sutton spoke to the state's health minister, Jenny Mikakos, who told him, 'Brett, whatever call you need to make, we'll back you completely.'

If you had to pinpoint the exact moment that the pandemic started in Australia in the minds of the public, it was a few hours later: about 10.00 am, Friday 13 March 2020, in Melbourne. Senior race official Henk van den Dungen was sitting in a course car idling at the start line of the Grand Prix circuit. To his left and right were towering stands and elevated corporate boxes. At any moment, he was going to switch on the flashing red lights on the roof of the vehicle and do a final lap of the Albert Park circuit before closing it off in preparation for the day's official racing schedule. Then came a call from race control. They told him, 'Don't close the track.' With just minutes to go, the Grand Prix had been officially called off. 'It was just such a disappointment, like a steep cliff, from being all excited and ready to go and then suddenly, nothing,' van den Dungen recalled. Instead of running the Grand Prix, he was sitting having a glass of red wine by lunchtime.

Until the last moment, it was almost business as usual inside the track, despite escalating rumours and media reports that the event would be cancelled. More than 300,000 spectators and a massive international contingent of media, drivers, and support staff were already in Melbourne waiting for the mega event to begin. Large crowds were pooling at the gates. Caterers had prepared the first meals of the day. About 850 volunteer race officials had already climbed onto buses and been distributed to dozens of locations around the circuit. Among them were marshals gripping a cluster of brightly coloured flags, and extrication teams in green overalls ready to rush in and pull drivers to safety.

Michael Smith, a director at Motorsport Australia and the man in charge of the race event, would describe the week preceding this day as like watching the tide come in. 'As the week progressed, it got closer and closer and just more intense,' he recalled. He realised they could be in trouble just a few days before the Formula One cars were due to begin qualifying, when US popstar Miley Cyrus pulled out of a bushfire-relief concert she was set to headline on Friday at the track, citing the 'current global health crisis'.

At six o'clock on Friday morning, Eugene Arocca, the chief executive of Motorsport Australia, switched on his radio as he drove to the track to hear news reports that two star drivers, Ferrari's Sebastian Vettel and Alfa Romeo's Kimi Raikkonen, had already boarded a plane and left Melbourne. 'It was the day that Australia woke up to Covid,' Arocca reflected later.

Around the same time, Brett Sutton was sitting on his couch at home when he burst into tears. He was exhausted, having worked through the night liaising with race officials and politicians. 'I'm not sure I can do this,' he told his wife, Kate, a leader in human rights and humanitarian aid. It was not merely the Grand Prix call that was weighing on his mind, but the ones he knew were to come.

'That [night] kind of laid out that there might be thousands of decisions like that in front of me,' Sutton told us. He said that his wife gave him 'an appropriate kick in the pants', and said that 'of course' he would be able to do it. In the early-morning conversations with the Australian Grand Prix Corporation, Sutton said race officials were ultimately willing to back what was necessary for public health. '[There were] lots of unhappy punters. I understand that … but again, in retrospect, it would have been the wrong decision to have let it go ahead,' he said.

Back in Sydney, West Australian premier Mark McGowan was eating an early breakfast with the Victorian premier, Daniel Andrews, who was talking about cancelling the Grand Prix. 'I just thought, *Wow*,' McGowan recalled, his eyes widening at the memory. 'I was sitting with him at breakfast and just thinking, *This is incredible*.' Andrews would front the media in Sydney soon after, telling them that if the race went ahead, it would be behind closed doors.

For weeks leading up to this moment, there had been speculation and debate about whether the Grand Prix should go ahead. Supercharging the question was the fact that Formula One giant Ferrari and tyre manufacturer Pirelli were based in the north of Italy, the country that for a time had led the global Covid-19 case toll. Ferrari and Pirelli staff had been allowed to enter Australia.

In a headline-making press conference one day before qualifying was due to begin, Lewis Hamilton, the sport's leading driver, said what many were thinking, telling reporters, 'I'm very very surprised that we are here … For me, it's really shocking that we are in this room.' Hamilton questioned why, at the same time that US president Donald Trump was shutting the borders to Europe, and the

NBA basketball league in the United States had been suspended, a motoring circus had come to town. When asked by a British journalist why he thought the race was still going on, he replied pointedly, 'Cash is king.' The headlines that day wrote themselves.

While Australia's borders were closed to visitors from China and then Iran and South Korea by the first week of March, an Italy travel ban wasn't announced by the prime minister until 11 March, by which time the Grand Prix teams had already arrived in Melbourne. That prompted questions about whether the federal government had been lobbied to delay the border closure to allow the event to proceed, although the federal health minister Greg Hunt told us it was the states' chief health officers, through the AHPPC, who were slow to recommend the action. On 4 March, the group had issued a statement saying they believed the government should now direct its focus towards domestic containment as 'border measures can no longer prevent importation of Covid-19'.

'Italy was falling apart,' Hunt said. 'The Italian Grand Prix teams were here, and the Grand Prix had not been called off. We think the order of things was that the Victorian political leadership was holding back the medical team, which was then holding back the borders.'

The news reports from Italy about lives being ended and upended provided a snapshot of the future for other Western countries. Schools were closed, and people were urged to stay at home. Funerals and weddings were cancelled. Italy's hospitals were overwhelmed to the point of collapse. Footage of gasping, feverish patients lining hospital corridors, exhausting and infecting doctors and nurses, was being projected across the world.

Morrison recalled watching one of the news reports late one night with his wife, Jenny, in an upstairs bedroom at The Lodge in Canberra. 'It was otherworldly,' he said. 'To see people on the ventilators, to see the chaos that was taking place. And this was a developed G7 economy with a health system—this was not in the third world.' Morrison said that he remarked to Jenny that he was worried about the fate of Australia's near-neighbour, Indonesia, which would see hundreds of thousands of excess deaths through the first two years of the pandemic.

Melbourne tradie Chris Miles, a motorsport fan, said that the most striking thing about Friday 13 March 2020 was that it was a perfect autumn day. It was too lovely, he said, for 'anything bad to happen'. As he hitched a ride on a packed tram to the Albert Park track that morning, rumours that the emerging virus could derail the Grand Prix was the hot topic of conversation, but few seemed genuinely concerned. Miles felt the other fans shared his view that this new disease would go in the same way of swine flu, SARS, and Ebola, where 'nothing really ever turned into anything'—at least anything that directly impacted his life. Yet the gates were, surprisingly, still shut when he reached the track's entry. 'I remember thinking this is so stupid; they don't want people to crowd, but then they have got these huge lines of people waiting.' Eventually, an official wielding a megaphone emerged to break the news. 'The [Australian Grand Prix Corporation] has been advised by Formula One that the Australian Grand Prix has been cancelled,' he said, looking nervous as he read off a mobile phone. 'Thank you again for your patience.'

Miles, a painter from Melbourne's north, who had been looking forward to a week off work and a busy weekend at the Grand Prix, experienced the first hint of a feeling that would grip Melburnians and other Australians during the years that followed: they didn't have anything to look forward to, and life seemed reduced to working, if you were lucky, and essential tasks. 'The hardest thing for me about the pandemic is I never had anything to look forward to,' he recalled. 'Something I'd really looked forward to for a long time was suddenly just taken away.'

Gathered together in Sydney, the nation's political leaders were already turning their minds to the question of what would come next. It was about 2.00 pm, and they had paused for lunch when, suddenly, the prime minister ordered all the advisers to leave the room. Left behind were Australia's six premiers and two chief ministers, plus Australia's chief medical officer, Brendan Murphy, who was about to reveal a dramatic escalation in the health advice.

'It really was a lightning bolt moment,' Queensland premier Annastacia Palaszczuk told us. Murphy had earlier briefed the leaders, gathered at a sports stadium in south-west Sydney, about Doherty modelling indicating that up to 150,000 Australians could die of the disease in an unmitigated, worst-case scenario. Steven Marshall, the South Australian premier, said it was clear to the leaders after the morning briefing that significant restrictions would need to be imposed in Australia, although this still seemed 'quite some time off'.

But as the politicians were meeting, so too were the nation's chief health officers in Canberra, led remotely by Murphy via video link. Cases of Covid-19 in Australia were suddenly surging, from just a handful each day to many dozens. Morrison said the phone of New South Wales premier Gladys Berejiklian was pinging with text messages from the state's chief health officer, Kerry Chant, confirming more and more cases.

Gunner's phone was vibrating, too. Medical supplies and body bags were being sent to remote Indigenous communities. Modelling that Gunner was receiving from the territory's medical team suggested that the territory would need at least 320 intensive-care beds. As of early 2020, it had just 24. Hospitals in the Northern Territory frequently ran beyond capacity, and treated a sparsely distributed population with rates of chronic disease among the highest in Australia. Even before the Covid pandemic, transfers of sick Territorians to other states were critical and commonplace. 'It was just horrifically alarming,' Gunner said. 'From that moment on, we basically said that the Northern Territory cannot afford to ever wait and have regrets, we have to go hard and early every time … We are literally talking about lives and the oldest living culture in the world. Incredibly vulnerable people. There were no do-overs.'

Of the 41 Covid-19 positive tests that would be returned in Australia on 13 March 2020, one belonged to home affairs minister

Peter Dutton. The former Queensland detective had woken up that morning with a temperature and a sore throat. Dutton had been in the United States several days earlier, where he had met with president Donald Trump's daughter Ivanka and US attorney-general William Barr. The next morning, Professor Paul Kelly, the nation's deputy chief medical officer, was startled to wake to a voicemail from the president's personal physician, wanting to know if the president had been a close contact of Dutton. He hadn't been, but Ivanka Trump and Barr would isolate as a precaution.

As the COAG meeting on 13 March had been nearing its close, Morrison was handed a note from Murphy. It revealed that the tenor and content of medical advice had changed: the health officials' group now urged immediate action. Morrison was reportedly less than pleased to be blindsided by what he saw as a rapid change in the position of the AHPPC. It was reported that the Victorian chief health officer, Brett Sutton, and Queensland's chief health officer, Jeannette Young, were particularly in favour of 'earlier and harder' restrictions.

'We were all like "What the hell just happened?"' Gunner recalled. 'My biggest takeaway from that was just the whiplash we all felt when the health advice suddenly did a 180.' Palaszczuk described the day as 'surreal', and said once the premiers had heard from Murphy, she told the leaders that there had to be 'some national consistency of messaging and national unity in how we responded'.

When the prime minister and premiers fronted the media at the end of the day, Morrison told journalists that a number of things had changed. One of them was growing evidence through the course of the day of a heightened community spread of coronavirus. Two significant announcements were also made. First, there would be an end to non-essential public gatherings of more than 500 people from the following Monday, triggering a wave of major event cancellations. The Sydney Royal Easter Show was cancelled for the first time since the Spanish Flu in 1919, along with the Melbourne International Comedy Festival. The second major announcement was the formation of a 'national cabinet' of federal, state, and territory leaders to deal with the coronavirus crisis. The national cabinet would meet weekly and be principally advised by the AHPPC, but would also receive counsel from others, including treasury boss Steven Kennedy and Reserve Bank of Australia governor Philip Lowe.

The seed of the idea for a national cabinet had been planted earlier that day, when Greg Hunt spoke to the Victorian president of the Australian Medical Association, Associate Professor Julian Rait, as he walked a six-kilometre route along the beach in Mount Martha and up into the Balcombe Estuary. Rait, a Melbourne ophthalmologist, had told Hunt about a university epidemiology-course essay he had written on the Spanish Flu. In 1919, the response to that pandemic had so fractured the relationship between the states and federal government that the fledgling federation had been threatened. Hunt repeated the conversation with Rait to the prime minister. He said the pair agreed that the goal was to have a single source of medical advice, and to bring the states into common alignment as much as possible, in the hope they could avoid similar quarrelling.

One hundred and one years earlier, Australia had delayed the arrival of the Spanish Flu by about six months, through its isolation and by quarantining maritime arrivals. The country's success in temporarily keeping the pneumonic influenza outbreak from making landfall was credited with saving many lives. However, tensions between the states and the Commonwealth quickly emerged in January 1919 when the first confirmed case of the virus, in a soldier, was detected in Victoria. The state delayed confirming the outbreak, and it subsequently spread into New South Wales and South Australia. It had been earlier agreed that the Commonwealth would be responsible for managing quarantine and proclaiming which states were infected, but after Victoria's delay in notifying the outbreak, the agreement was irreparably damaged. Instead, the states ended up organising their own border controls.

The responses varied, but schools, churches, theatres, and pubs were closed in many parts of Australia. Globally, the second and third waves of the Spanish Flu killed a surprisingly large number of young and healthy people, in addition to those who had already perished in their millions during the World War I. Victory celebrations for the war, which ended just as the flu pandemic began, were delayed as a result of the contagion.

In 2020, the national cabinet was instantly busy and, for some of the time, harmonious. 'My one overarching takeaway from national cabinet was that everyone in the room, regardless of their political persuasion, was there to do the right thing,' said Peter Gutwein, the Liberal premier of Australia's smallest state, Tasmania. 'They were a good bunch of people we worked with, and we had one aim in mind, which is to save as many lives as possible.'

Steven Marshall, then South Australia's Liberal premier, said there were weeks that he and the other leaders were meeting via national cabinet two to three times a week. 'I think we had 58 meetings in 100 weeks,' Marshall recalled. 'Compare that to COAG, which used to be held once or twice per year. So we had the equivalent of 30 or 40 years worth of COAG meetings.'

The Labor chief minister of the Australian Capital Territory, Andrew Barr, made similar but more pointed observations. He said that national cabinet was sometimes marred with tensions, disputes, and 'chips on shoulders' that made him feel like he was 'back in the colonies' when Australia's six British colonies united to form the Commonwealth of Australia in 1901.

'It's no secret that Premier Berejiklian and Morrison didn't get on particularly well. It's no secret that Berejiklian and Annastacia Palaszczuk weren't the best of mates. It's no secret that at times the federal government was at absolute war with Daniel Andrews,' Barr said. '[There was] no love lost between Western Australia and New South Wales at various points.'

However, Barr said he also believed the federation generally stood up well and that national cabinet often showed its worth. 'It wasn't as if we just spent 67 meetings being narky with each other. There was a lot of cooperation, and hours and hours and hours of meetings, and a constant stream of advice,' he said. 'I think the fact that there was the full spectrum of political ideology represented in the room … brought the Australian response more back to the sensible centre most of the time.'

Some of those working at the frontline of Australia's pandemic response hadn't had a summer break before the pandemic, as the nation was consumed by the bushfires. Now they were working every day, from dawn and well into the night, sometimes up to 20 hours at a time. This would continue for almost two years. Many spoke of regular exercise as a vital mental and physical lifeline.

As a federal politician with a major portfolio, Greg Hunt was accustomed to sleeping about six hours a night. In the fervid early days of the pandemic, he survived on about four. When he finally got to bed, he'd often fall asleep with a book still in his hand. The father of two had been a committed runner before Covid. He switched to walking during the pandemic, using the time to read and respond to hundreds of text messages. They came from colleagues, state politicians, media, interest groups, friends looking for advice, and even ordinary constituents of his Mornington Peninsula electorate. He called the process 'clearing'. As the sun seeped over the horizon, he would text and walk, and call people.

But Hunt grew to loathe his phone and the constant stream of incoming correspondence, estimating he was receiving and replying to about 600 to 1,000 text messages a day. 'Life was work and exercise,' he said. 'The thing that missed out was family, even when you were based at home, if you were [getting through] 500 to 1,000 messages on the weekend, there's still no time for them,' he said. 'That was probably the worst of all, being physically present but not intellectually or emotionally present.'

In South Australia, the state's chief public health officer, Professor Nicola Spurrier, read *The Plague*, a novel by French philosopher Albert Camus, first published in 1947. In the book, the bubonic plague sweeps through a town in Algeria. Authorities are slow to take action. The hospital is quickly overrun; homes are quarantined; the town is sealed off; and there is a shortage of 'plague serum'. 'I found that very, very interesting,' said Spurrier. 'It was like my life was being played out.'

The head of epidemiology of the Doherty Institute, Jodie McVernon, was watching the dystopian television drama *Years and Years*, set between 2019 and 2034, which imagines a monkey flu pandemic, death camps, and Donald Trump winning a second term as president. She found it strangely comforting. 'At that point, I would wake up in the morning and think, *Oh, I have had this terrible nightmare,*' she recalled. But then the realisation would dawn on her that it wasn't her imagination—it was real life. Later on, McVernon, a mother of two teenagers, remembers a note being slipped under the door of the 'good room' where she was busy on video calls. Her children, who were studying from home in bayside Melbourne because their schools were closed, were asking if they could book half an hour with her.

Western Australia's chief health officer, Dr Andy Robertson, said that during March 2020 the AHPPC was working seven days a week. He was often back in his office until ten o'clock at night. The early mornings were even earlier for Robertson, who was operating on Western Australian time. One morning, he woke up to find that he had missed a meeting that had happened while he was sleeping. 'They'd run it at 8.30 in the morning, and I politely pointed out that it was 5.30 in the morning here.' Around this time, the AHPPC began advising the community that they should have no more than one person per four square metres in closed spaces. Professor James McCaw, who is six foot three, remembers standing up in a meeting room as the public health officials were workshopping this rule, and spinning around in a circle with his arms outstretched. Then Brendan Murphy stood up, too, and they made sure their hands weren't touching. 'That's where the four-square metre rule came from,' McCaw explained. 'It was a practical way for people to understand how to keep a safer distance from each other.'

As the local outbreak continued to grow, the nation's top public health officials began making their toughest recommendations yet. A few days earlier, a call had been made to require anyone arriving in Australia from overseas to isolate at home or at a hotel for 14 days—a devastating blow for the nation's tourism industry. On 17 March, they were talking about denying people the most important thing in their life: access to their family. Aged-care residents would have their outings cancelled, and visitors restricted to two people a day. They were not allowed to see their young relatives at all, unless they had an exemption. The normally sacrosanct ANZAC Day ceremonies, due to be held the following month, were to be cancelled.

'That meeting was tough,' recalled McCaw. 'There were a lot of emotions.' Underlying the intensity of the pressure that these previously anonymous public servants faced, McCaw said there were numerous times in the pandemic that a chief health officer was brought to tears during meetings. Once, a chief health officer became so stressed that they were incapable of thinking clearly for a while. 'They were flipping between looking like a deer in the headlights and starting to say some pretty silly stuff,' he said. 'The gravity of the situation almost broke, or briefly did break, one of the chief health officers. [They] had to get back on their game. And they did just minutes later, and they continue to do excellent work.'

On the evening of 17 March, a small delegation of AHPPC members made their way to dinner at a restaurant in Canberra to reflect and to decompress. As he looked around the busy bar, McCaw said he felt like the little group was carrying a secret. 'We knew we had just put down on paper things that were going to define the lives of Australians for the next few years, and no one else knew about it,' he said. The statement prepared by the AHPPC that day included a graph showing that while Australia had one of the lowest rates of cases of Covid-19 compared to similar countries, it was also much earlier in its outbreak. In fact, Australia was following a route closest to the trajectory of the UK, France, Germany, and the US.

Australian doctors were terrified about what might just be around the corner. In petitions, thousands were urging the government to follow several European countries into an immediate national lockdown of schools, churches, gyms, pubs, bars, and theatres. 'Many of us are in contact with colleagues in Italy, Spain, and France and they are begging us to learn from their mistakes,' said a letter from doctors to the prime minister. However, the position of the AHPPC was that school closures were not yet necessary, and could result in close to a third of Australia's health staff being unable to work. The group also argued against a short-term shutdown of the nation. 'There is no way that we can lock down society and make everyone stay home, and then in a month's time undo that, because the virus will just flare up again without any real long-term benefit,' Brendan Murphy said. 'We have to have sustainable measures.'

At Melbourne's Austin Hospital, the intensive-care director, Associate Professor Stephen Warrillow, said there was a spreadsheet being drawn up, containing the contact details of every living health-care worker who had ever worked at the hospital, should they be called on to help. He discussed whether garbage bags could be used if the hospital ran out of protective gowns. Plans were drawn up to increase intensive-care capacity by 400 per cent, and potentially beyond. For the first time in its history, the emergency department was split in two. The downstairs emergency triage centre became a unit for suspected cases of Covid-19. An upstairs ward on level three was converted into a Covid-19 isolation area. The door to the ward was firmly sealed shut, and there was a bright-yellow sign on the window: 'Covid-19 room. Quarantine area. No visitors allowed.' Frontline staff changed into their scrubs at work. When their shift ended, they would leave their scrubs to be cleaned at the hospital. Many were so concerned about infecting their families when they got home from work that they left their shoes at the door and immediately stripped down, soaking their clothes in a bucket of hot soapy water.

It was a frightening and confusing time. Despite the official health advice, school attendances plunged in many states. Messages spreading misinformation about lockdowns and the virus were shared widely on social media. Overnight, people lost their jobs and businesses. Australia's national airline, Qantas, stood down 20,000 workers—two-thirds of its workforce—without pay. The company's chief executive, Alan Joyce, argued it was a case of 'survival of the fittest'. It was predicted that house prices could plunge by 20 per cent or more. People started hoarding food and medicines again. Buying limits were extended to other basic items: pasta, flour, rice, paper towels, tissues, and hand sanitiser. 'Stop hoarding,' pleaded Morrison. 'I can't be more blunt about it. Stop it. It is not sensible, it is not helpful, and it has been one of the most disappointing things I have seen in Australian behaviour in response to this crisis. That is not who we are as a people.' Special shopping hours were introduced for the elderly and vulnerable in an attempt to shield them from other rushing shoppers.

It was around this time that 2GB radio personality Ben Fordham recorded an entire radio show that would never see the light of day. The host of Sydney's highest-rating breakfast show had been staying in Melbourne to film the television show *Australian Ninja Warrior*. One day, his co-host, Rebecca Maddern, didn't turn up, having been placed into isolation because she had been in contact with entertainment reporter Richard Wilkins, who by then had coronavirus. Then English cricketer Freddie Flintoff, who was also part of the show's cast, made the decision to fly back to the UK, worried that the borders would shut and he wouldn't be able to get home.

Fordham decided to record a back-up show just in case there was a shutdown of the Melbourne CBD and he wasn't able to make his way into the 3AW offices in Docklands, where he was broadcasting at the time. He compared the moment to the infamous video of far-right politician Pauline Hanson when she declared: 'Fellow Australians, if you are seeing me now, it means I have been murdered.' (The video was leaked, and Hanson was not murdered.)

'It was literally me saying, "If you're listening to this show, it means that I am unable to broadcast at the moment due to coronavirus",'

Fordham said. After seeing pictures of long queues of the newly unemployed snaking outside the Centrelink offices, Fordham also went and withdrew $5,000 cash from a bank near the Melbourne radio studio. 'I gave it to my executive producer, Zac McLean, and I said, "Stuff this in your bag", and he looked at me like, "What the fuck are you talking about?", and I said, "Mate, I don't know what's going on,"' he remembered. 'It doesn't make sense, but when you're in the middle of something that you've never experienced before, you do find yourself making some pretty bizarre judgement calls.'

Fordham could only remember one show before the pandemic that he had dedicated entirely to a single topic, on the day of the Christchurch mosque shootings in 2019, when 51 people were massacred by an Australian white supremacist. But for months and months in many newsrooms across Australia, it felt like coronavirus was the only story that mattered, and it consumed newspaper headlines and television news bulletins like no issue this century.

Fordham said his producers would challenge him early on to cover other topics, but he would reply to them, 'Why? Are your friends talking about anything else?' He would field questions from listeners about the virus and the rules that had been hastily introduced in the face of rising cases. 'We were desperate to know whether things were better or worse. How many cases? How many were in hospital? What the latest rules were. What our vaccine levels were. What was happening in other parts of the country and the world ... Every day, every hour, every minute, every second, there was nothing else in town that anyone was interested in.'

CHAPTER FIVE

The Ruby Princess

It was a Saturday night on the Ruby Princess, somewhere off the coast of New Zealand. The massive cruise liner was heaving with merry guests. Champagne was fizzing. Cutlery was clinking. Shows were about to begin. But buried in the bulk of the floating hotel, a few passengers weren't joining in the merriment. Tony Londero, an explosives technician from the small town of Quirindi in New South Wales, was nursing a headache. Back in his small cabin with his wife, Kerry, he flicked on the television. A news bulletin flashed up, and a reporter announced that hundreds of people in Italy had died of coronavirus.

It had been six days since the Ruby Princess had left Sydney Harbour, on 8 March, and the 62-year-old had been busy with an eclectic mix of activities catering for the mostly grey-haired guests. There had been Rod Stewart and ABBA tributes. He had joined choir sessions and had partnered with a woman in her 80s who was travelling with her sister at several line and Latin dancing classes. However, when Londero and his wife gathered with their close friends Paul and Linda Cheyne in Skywalkers Nightclub later that same Saturday night, he told them that he no longer wanted to go to any shows or mix with people. 'I said I feel we should be really careful because I wasn't feeling 100 per cent. What I saw on the news was scaring me. I don't know whether they thought I was panicking, but they took the advice on board, and we just kept a very low profile after that.'

He was very right to be worried. As became apparent to New South Wales authorities much too late, the boat had an unwelcome stowaway. The undetected Covid-19 outbreak on the ship was to become the largest superspreading event detected in Australia. Of the 1,682 Australian passengers, 663 people—roughly 40 per cent—ended up testing positive for Covid-19. Of the crew, at least 191 caught the virus. There were another 965 guests who came from overseas. Because all their infections couldn't be traced, the total number of passengers who caught Covid-19 on the Ruby Princess will never be known. Many of the passengers were extremely vulnerable to the disease, being older, and, during these formative days of the pandemic, unvaccinated.

This voyage and the events that followed was the first big scandal of the pandemic in Australia, attracting an enormous level of scrutiny. The disaster quickly sparked a special inquiry, a criminal investigation, an apology from New South Wales premier Gladys Berejiklian, and the beginnings of a class action against the ship's owner and operator, Princess Cruise Lines and Carnival. Why the state authorities allowed hundreds of passengers—120 of them symptomatic and none of them Covid-tested—to disembark from the ship at Sydney during a global pandemic has been subject to intense review. Years later, questions were still being asked about why the ship was allowed to sail at all.

On 15 March, the Ruby Princess had just left Napier, on the North Island of New Zealand, when the Australian government announced a 30-day ban on cruise ships docking in Australia. An exception was given to ships that started sailing directly back to Australia before midnight that day, which included the Ruby Princess. Instead of travelling on to Tauranga, Auckland, and the Bay of Islands, it made a U-turn and a beeline back across the Tasman Sea.

The next day, a note was slid quietly under the door of the Londeros' cabin, instructing anyone with a temperature to report to the sickbay. Still feeling unwell, Londero made his way down to the medical centre, where the ship's doctors examined him. There was something straining his heart, he said, to the point there were signs he was having a heart attack. But there was no rushing him to an emergency room, specialists, and a cardiac lab. Instead, he had to wait it out with the medical staff on board for days more. A coronavirus swab was taken, but it wasn't possible to process it on board.

More than a month earlier, two senior New South Wales public health officials, Dr Leena Gupta and Dr David Durrheim, had pushed for special procedures that would have made a major difference at this juncture. They had argued that Covid-19 samples should be tested before cruise ship passengers were allowed to disembark in New South Wales, even if that meant putting the tests on a helicopter and flying them to a lab ahead of time. Durrheim had warned that the cruise ships were a 'petri-dish environment' for the virus to spread, and that once passengers had disembarked, it would already be too late to rein any outbreak in. These comments weren't just an educated guess. At the top of their minds was a continuing coronavirus drama involving another ship from the same fleet as the Ruby Princess, the Diamond Princess. For a time, that liner hosted the largest known coronavirus outbreak in the world, outside China.

At least 164 Australians were quarantined on the Diamond Princess in February as it was moored in Yokohama, Japan, with the long lenses of the world's media trained upon it. Passengers were confined to their cabins, some of them without windows or a balcony, for two weeks before an Australian Medical Assistance Team and a Qantas plane was dispatched to retrieve them. Australia's chief nursing and midwifery officer, Professor Alison McMillan, was working in Canberra when she received a call giving her two hours' notice to pack her backpack and get ready to fly to Japan. By the next morning, she and the team were in mini-buses whipping past a thronging delegation of international press and across a vast wharf, armed with a map showing the location of the rooms of the Australian passengers.

The Diamond Princess was impressive, a floating skyscraper. 'I'd never seen anything like it,' said McMillan. 'It was towering, like a giant building above you.' Inside, workers in white Hazmat suits were a strange sight wandering through the gilded lobbies. The Australian team went from door to door, explaining the plan to fly passengers back to the Howard Springs quarantine centre just out of Darwin. McMillan was paired with an infection-control nurse from Ballarat, and was allocated a group of guests. She remembers telling one couple that they would be back to see them later in the day to take them back to the airport. 'As they closed the door, we could hear them whooping and squealing with excitement. They knew they were going home.'

Not everyone could make the flight. A man who had been on his honeymoon had Covid-19 and had to remain behind. McMillan said she generally found the Australian passengers healthy and in good spirits, but, as is often the case with coronavirus, the disease can brew mildly before worsening suddenly. One of the Australians who had been on board the Diamond Princess was Western Australian tourism industry stalwart James Kwan, who had founded the Wel-Travel travel agency in 1988. He spent two weeks in Howard Springs after catching Covid, and was pictured walking off a flight when he arrived back home in Perth in February. But his condition deteriorated, and the next month the 78-year-old died in hospital. He was Australia's first coronavirus death.

It was a few weeks later, in the early hours of 19 March 2020, that the Ruby Princess returned to Circular Quay. As other passengers slept soundly on board, with the green-blue water of Sydney Harbour lapping gently below, Tony Londero left the boat strapped onto an ambulance gurney. The two paramedics who led him away wore what was to become a familiar uniform of the pandemic: yellow gowns, blue gloves, and face masks. The mystery of what was causing Londero's symptoms was solved when he tested positive for Covid-19 at the Royal Prince Alfred Hospital. In an isolation room, he began to experience hallucinations so vivid he said it was like being in a time machine. They carried him back to his childhood, where he walked the streets of Bourke, in outback New South Wales, heard people talk, and smelled the warm country air.

'Even though I had the logic to know I was in big trouble, it was also so incredible to be back there. It was just so crystal clear, my memory.' It was when he was in that room, often left alone, that he experienced the worst of the disease, struggling to breathe or too weak or confused to press the emergency button. When he finally started to improve, it felt like his feet were catching fire. The grandfather of seven said he was later told that this was because his extremities had been shutting down, and the burning was the feeling of the blood returning to his feet. He ran them under cold water.

Ten days after he was stretchered off the Ruby Princess, still so weak he was unable to walk properly, he was discharged to a nearby virtual hospital, a repurposed hotel. Food was left outside the door. Nurses were able to remotely check most vital signs, and they popped in wearing PPE once a day to check his blood pressure. Also staying at the facility was his wife, Kerry, although they weren't able to see each other until a couple of days into his stay, when a fire alarm went off. Londero, who had already been through so much, thought darkly that he'd made it this far, and now he was going to burn. Instead, he found himself evacuated onto the street, where husband and wife were at last reunited on the footpath. They looked like an odd pair the next day, when they squeezed themselves into an Uber wearing plastic gowns, masks, and gloves, finally on their way home. The driver didn't question their strange outfits.

On the morning that the Ruby Princess returned to Sydney, Blue Mountains retirees Kathleen and Richard Humphrey had been sitting under a large fig tree when their daughter, Louise Butlin, picked them up from Circular Quay. Butlin was running late because her mother had told her that she expected to be delayed in disembarking the boat while coronavirus testing took place.

'I thought, *Oh my God, they're going to be there for hours,*' she said. 'But then at nine o'clock in the morning she rings me and says, "We're off the ship." I was shocked, and I hadn't even left home yet.'

The Humphreys, both in their 80s, lived in a house dubbed 'the love shack' that adjoined the home of their daughter, Louise, and her husband, Scott, in a bushy suburb called Blaxlands Ridge near Richmond, north-west of Sydney. Louise Butlin and her mother were best friends and the only women in a household of boys—their husbands, and Butlin's four sons. Although Kathleen Humphrey was 81, Butlin said she had the energy of a woman a decade younger. She was always beautifully dressed, loyal, and loved her family and friends, who loved her back just as fiercely.

Butlin and her husband had both tried talking her parents out of going on the cruise, as news of the fate of the Diamond Princess hit the headlines in Australia, but to no avail. Butlin said they were reassured by text messages in the lead-up to their departure and her mother's firm faith that Princess Cruises wouldn't put them in any danger. 'She had been on so many cruises with them,' Butlin explained. 'She just thought they were the ultimate; she idolised Princess Cruises. She said, "Princess Cruises would not let us on that ship if there was Covid on it."'

For ten days after the Humphreys arrived home, everything seemed fine. Butlin had been checking in with her parents as they waited out a 14-day quarantine period. Every day, she walked across the courtyard that separated their properties and popped her head in the door. Then, one morning, she discovered her mother 'deathly pale'. 'She was just sitting there—she hadn't eaten, she hadn't drunk anything. She was shivering. She was in a dressing gown, and it wasn't really that cold.'

Kathleen Humphrey spent about six weeks in the intensive-care unit of the Nepean Hospital, on the suburban fringe of Sydney. For much of the time, her family were unable to visit her due to infection-control protocols. All they were able to do was call in and have a one-sided conversation. 'A couple of times, she was semi-awake, and the nurses would say she's nodding her head, or she's crying. When the grandkids rang up, she would smile, so at least she knew we were talking to her,' Butlin said.

'Eventually … she would go into a normal ICU bed, but she was still intubated, which meant she couldn't talk, and she was so weak she couldn't even lift her arms. They gave her a letterboard thing to try to spell out words, but it was no good; she couldn't really do that. So we would just sit there and talk. My dad would say something stupid, and she'd roll her eyes.'

They hoped for a miracle when she was given a tracheostomy, and she was able to say her daughter's name, Louise, through the speaking valve in her throat, in a Darth Vadar-like voice. But around this time, a doctor showed Butlin an X-ray of her mother's lungs, all clouded in white. 'The black in the picture is the bad part and the white is the good part,' the doctor said, before realising in horror she had explained it wrong. The *white* was the bad part, and there was barely any black left. 'That's when it really hit me that my mum was going to die and there was no hope,' Butlin said.

In Kathleen Humphrey's final hours, they played her favourite music, Rod Stewart songs, and a chaplain from the hospital said a prayer. 'The worst thing was they brought her out of a coma a little bit, so we could talk to her, and when we were saying the Lord's Prayer at the end, she was trying to mouth words,' Butlin said. 'That really killed us, because she was religious and she did believe in heaven. She then knew she was going to die. I just hoped she was comforted, she had us there, and the music was playing. All we could do was hold her hand, and that's what we did.'

Butlin said her mother's doctor also cried at the end. The same doctor had been ringing her contacts across the world to confer on the best-known methods of treating Covid-19 patients, and she gave the family two knitted red love hearts, donated by someone she knew in Ireland. Kathleen kept one with her, at the very end.

At a time when coronavirus still carried a heavy stigma, the death notice in the *Sydney Morning Herald* for Kathleen Humphrey honouring the 'loved nana' defiantly noted her 'brave battle after The Ruby Princess'. Louise Butlin firmly believed that if it wasn't for decisions made by the cruise company, her mother would have had years ahead of her. 'She should not be dead,' she said. 'I believe that there were just a whole lot of executives sitting around a table going, "We'll get one more cruise in, it's worth the risk." ... 'It's terrible to say, but I feel like they murdered her like that. That's how angry I am about it. That ship should have never left.'

By late March 2020, cases linked to the ship were in their hundreds. Members of the ship's crew, still confined to the ship, were among the sick. Despite this, the Ruby Princess was initially ordered out of Australian waters. New South Wales police commissioner Mick Fuller told the operators of six ships off the state's coast that it was 'time to go back to your port of origin'.

Dean Summers, who was the national coordinator of the International Transport Workers' Federation during the pandemic, was angry when he talked about how the crew on the Ruby Princess, and other ships, were treated. Summers explained that the Ruby Princess was flying under the flag of the Bahamas. It is what is described as a flag of convenience, a practice often used to avoid tax or bypass workplace regulations. 'The Bahamas government weren't taking any responsibility, and we wouldn't expect them to,' Summers said. 'If that ship was full of Australians, they wouldn't have dreamed of treating those people like they did.'

Concern from the Australian public helped broker an alternative arrangement that saw the Ruby Princess granted a safe haven of sorts at Port Kembla, south of Sydney. Summers believes they were put there to be out of sight. Instead, they were met in a virtual embrace by the local Illawarra community. Along with the local Mission to Seafarers, they provided a reported 1,200 care packages for the stranded crew before hundreds were repatriated to their home countries and the ship finally left Australian waters on 23 April.

At least 28 passengers on the Ruby Princess—20 from Australia and eight from the United States — lost their lives after becoming infected with coronavirus. The outbreak first leached out unnoticed, as passengers harbouring the virus dispersed around Australia and the world. The investigations that followed noted that the procedures surrounding the Ruby Princess disembarkation on 19 March differed greatly from the voyage that directly preceded it. That earlier journey, another round trip between Australia and New Zealand, between 24 February and 8 March, had been declared as carrying a 'medium risk' of harbouring the disease. There was particular concern about two UK passengers who had tested negative for influenza, but who had a cough and a runny nose, and had recently visited Singapore. Before the ship arrived back in Sydney, an announcement had been made for everyone with a 'travel history of concern' or respiratory symptoms to present themselves to the dining room for screening.

A senior epidemiologist who boarded the ship, Kelly-Anne Ressler, said that the health team were 'shocked' to see many more people than listed on the ship's log with respiratory symptoms — 240 of the 366 people in the dining room. Four of them with unexplained fever, severe coughs, and systemic illness were tested for Covid, as well as three crew members who had fevers. Dr Vicky Sheppeard, the deputy director of the local health unit, who made the decision to test the passengers and crew, said the swabs were precautionary, as not all of these persons fitted the epidemiological criteria for a suspected Covid case. Once they came back negative, the next round of passengers — including the Londeros and the Humphreys — were allowed to board. The New South Wales police commissioner later said an infected crew member was most likely responsible for the subsequent outbreak.

It might follow that similar testing protocols would have occurred when the Ruby Princess returned again ten days later, arriving in a nation that had changed at warp speed since it had last berthed. A global pandemic had been declared. Non-essential gatherings of 100 people had just been banned, and ANZAC Day ceremonies had been cancelled. Here was a ship on which thousands of people had spent days mingling and dining together freely without a thought for social distancing. Yet the Ruby Princess on its return was declared low-risk. Part of this decision can be traced back to the fact that the expert panel making the call had slightly outdated information that under-counted the number of people on the ship with an influenza-like illness. You could also argue that there was a failure of common sense.

Commissioner Bret Walker, in his final report on the Ruby Princess, argued that receiving the Covid-19 test results before letting passengers leave the ship was 'rudimentary and very important'. Not only was there a real possibility that the virus was on board, but, if that was the case, all those on the ship would have been considered close contacts, he said. It took almost 30 hours for the results to be returned from the Ruby Princess. New South Wales Health also initially provided incorrect advice that passengers could catch flights home overseas and interstate if they were well, despite the require-ment in force at the time for cruise-ship passengers to immediately quarantine in local accommodation for 14 days.

It was estimated that another 176 people caught Covid-19 as a result of the unfettered disembarkation, including a deadly outbreak at the North West Regional Hospital in Tasmania, where a Ruby Princess passenger was the suspected source. Although it comes as little comfort for those harmed by these infections, it could have been far worse, with most of the cases linked to the ship still confined to those who had been on board.

CHAPTER SIX

Lights off

Legendary sports commentator Bruce McAvaney was struggling to find his groove. It was the season-opening match of the Australian Football League, and the Melbourne Cricket Ground (MCG) should have been teeming with more than 80,000 fans. Instead, the stands were almost bare, and goals were being kicked without a roar of celebration. It felt more like a training drill, not the curtain raiser for the nation's most popular sports league. 'You felt like a single sentence was rebounding in your ears,' McAvaney told us from his home in Adelaide, where his brown-and-white dog, Frankie, sat by his feet. 'I found it quite difficult to get rhythm and to feel as if I had real substance in the sound of my voice, and what I was saying as a result.'

The day before the opening match, between reigning premiers Richmond and their hometown rivals Carlton, the AFL had made an unprecedented decision to proceed with the new season without crowds. During the Spanish Flu pandemic of 1919, the Victorian Football League had been allowed to play a full 18 rounds with spectators, even as schools and theatres were closed. A century later, football administrators had been left with little choice — either to play before empty stadiums, or not at all, following the ban on mass public gatherings. This game on the evening of 19 March 2020 still stands as having provided one of the most profound shocks of the pandemic. While by this point the major-events industry in Australia had come to a halt, the crowdless game played at 'the G', the largest stadium in the Southern Hemisphere, was intensely symbolic of the moment, and of how very far life had veered from normal.

McAvaney stood near the centre of the vast stadium to begin his opening address to viewers. 'This time last year, there were 85,000 fans at the 'G for the traditional season opener,' he began, as the camera zoomed in. 'Who could have imagined at the start of the 2020 season there would be empty stands, and, dare I say it, a very quiet stadium? It's going to feel different tonight. It's going to sound different tonight. We wish all you fans were in here with us, but we know, all of us, that there are more important matters at play right now.'

During a usual prime-time football game, the noise of the crowd would be playing quite loudly through the headphones of McAvaney and the other presenters in the Channel Seven commentary box. Its absence that night was starving McAvaney of the oxygen that drove his commentary. 'It lifts you and gives you a bit more oomph in your voice, and a bit more timbre, so to speak,' he explained. 'I couldn't find that, I couldn't find that little bit extra.' The veteran caller, by now in his late 60s, was well known for his meticulous preparation and work ethic, but by his own lofty standards at least, he was falling short. At the end of the match, McAvaney found himself uncomfortable at the prospect of more matches, possibly finals, being played in the same conditions. He thought, *This is not going to be what I've lapped up for 30 years or 20 years.*

There would be more upheaval to come. Just three days after this Thursday-night game, the AFL women's season was cancelled, and the men's was suspended for more than two months. League chief Gillon McLachlan said the decision had been made because of Australia's worsening Covid situation and the decision by some state governments to close their borders. The league, whose top players are paid in excess of $1 million a year, stood down most of its staff. Even assistant coaches were placed on unpaid leave. The players took a temporary pay cut, and Australians got accustomed to a new word: 'furlough'.

A little-known fact about the 2020 AFL season is that McAvaney spent the majority of it anchoring games in a small conference room in Adelaide at the local headquarters of Seven. McAvaney stood at a lectern, stacked with piles of paper and a few highlighters, the boardroom table a tangle of cords, plugged into broadcasting equipment. The lack of a crowd in the first couple of AFL games had been so disconcerting and unpopular that a decision was made to play a soundtrack of 'canned' crowd noise during subsequent games. 'We don't usually like fake, but it was beneficial to a broadcaster, and I think it was certainly beneficial to the people at home,' McAvaney said.

March in Australia in 2020 was marked by cancellations, job losses, rising infections, and the fear of more to come. Australian governments busied themselves preparing for the worst. Federal health minister Greg Hunt described setting up a new telehealth system within ten days, so Australians could consult with their doctors without leaving the house. 'We could see what was happening in Italy and Spain and France and New York, in particular,' he said. 'Their primary health systems were collapsing, their aged-care systems were collapsing, and the hospital systems were collapsing. Doctors were dying, nurses were dying, and they were walking off the job.'

It felt like a last hurrah when thousands of people descended on Bondi Beach on 20 March, soaking up the late-autumn sunshine in defiance of authorities' requests not to gather in large numbers. One guilty Sydneysider interviewed by American television network CBS, her hair still soggy from a swim, said that the world was probably looking at Australia and thinking what a massive mistake it was making.

Come Sunday, the New South Wales, Victorian, and Australian Capital Territory governments announced that their states would be closing all non-essential services within the coming 48 hours, blind-siding prime minister Scott Morrison, who worried that the shut-down plans lacked detail.

The chief minister of the Australian Capital Territory, Andrew Barr, felt Morrison wanted to stay at the helm of the pandemic deci-sion-making. 'That Sunday was the first time that premiers and chief ministers pushed back in a substantial way,' Barr said. New South Wales premier Gladys Berejiklian and Victorian premier Daniel Andrews were perhaps at the more concerned end of the spectrum, he said, given the heightened risk of coronavirus taking off in the large cosmopolitan cities of Sydney and Melbourne. Almost 100 new cases had been detected in New South Wales the day before, and 67 in Victoria. Barr said, given that the Australian Capital Territory, the small landlocked home of the nation's capital, was entirely enclosed within the state of New South Wales, it was always going to be at a heightened risk of suffering an outbreak from its larger neighbour.

That evening, after a quickly convened national cabinet meeting, Morrison detailed a series of measures that it had been agreed would apply across Australia. Pubs, clubs, cinemas, casinos, indoor sporting venues, churches, and mosques would close by midday Monday. Restaurants and cafés would be restricted to takeaway only. Victoria had decided to end the school term a couple of days early, and when term two rolled around a few weeks later, most states, with a few exceptions, encouraged or required parents to keep their children at home.

As thousands of businesses were forced to shut, lines hundreds of metres long spilled outside welfare offices. When Michael Gunner, the Northern Territory's chief minister, watched a television inter-view with a distraught man standing in a queue in Darwin applying for unemployment benefits for the first time, he had flashbacks to his own father. Gunner grew up on the rough side of Alice Springs in public housing, often couch surfing with his family. 'I could picture my old man in that line,' he said. 'I thought, *We've done this to him*. I'd cost him his job, and at that point in time his pride. I was desperately hoping that I was saving his life, and therefore I could justify it to myself.'

Morrison said it was these queues that were front of mind when he and his ministers devised a wage-subsidy scheme they hoped would avoid a mass layoff of workers from the businesses no longer functioning. 'What we had to do is come up with something that had to deal with, essentially, five million people. Now, on its best day, social security cannot deal with that volume.' The solution was JobKeeper. Instead of asking millions to join the welfare lines, possibly never to be rehired, affected businesses were given $1,500 to pay each worker every fortnight. The payment, which lasted six months before being reduced, effectively doubled the welfare rate for the unemployed, which people had long argued was insufficient to keep families out of poverty anyway.

JobKeeper was not without its controversies. Billions were paid to companies that would go on to record an upturn in their profits. Yet the scheme was credited with saving about 800,000 jobs. In a 2023 interview, Morrison said it was hard for him to pay for a coffee most of the time. 'People want to offer me one, to say thank you … I think there is a very quiet appreciation for all those things out there.'

As more than 300 new coronavirus cases were recorded on 24 March, Morrison returned to the lectern in Canberra to announce a new and rambling list of things that Australians could and couldn't do. Only five people could attend weddings; no more than ten mourners could attend funerals. The shutdown was extended to brothels, tattoo parlours, open house inspections, play centres, beauty salons, and yoga and barre studios. In a gaffe of sorts, Morrison stumbled over the word barre, admitting he wasn't sure what the ballet-inspired exercise was or how to pronounce it, before taking an unsuccessful punt on 'barr-ay'. Morrison brings up his error when reflecting on these evening press conferences, this time nailing the pronunciation: 'bar'.

'I'm now well versed in this athletic pursuit. But that really showed how detailed this thing had to get,' he said. Morrison and

Hunt were concerned that when Victoria and New South Wales jumped ahead of national cabinet, announcing a shutdown on 22 March, they would cause confusion and undermine essential industries. They wanted the states to provide a clear and detailed list explaining exactly what would and wouldn't shut. 'They were going to move to ... a short list of permissible activities, but that would have led to hospital closures, possibly electricity failures,' Hunt said.

Victorian premier Daniel Andrews told journalist Patrick Carlyon he believed that if Victoria had waited a week to act, the virus would have spread beyond control. 'You've got a moment, and you've got a real sense that if you don't do something now, you won't get this moment back.'

The Australian Capital Territory chief minister, Andrew Barr, said, 'Had it just been left to the Commonwealth and the prime minister, I don't know if those decisions would have been made on that day.'

Often in the Covid pandemic, quick and decisive action was required. Sometimes that necessitated making policy on the run. Morrison remembers waking on the morning of 25 March to find his phone filled with messages about a rule he had announced the evening before, capping haircuts at 30 minutes. As Morrison soon learnt, most women's hair appointments span several hours. 'One look at me will tell you I don't have a great deal of knowledge of these things, and frankly the blokes around the room didn't,' he said, starting to laugh. 'I got onto [New South Wales Premier Gladys Berejiklian] and said, "I think we're going to have to change this."'

By late March, Melbourne's office towers were filled with empty desks and lonely swivel chairs. The hotels had cleared out, too, their beds stripped down and their corridors silent. As the hotel industry contemplated financial ruin, Victorian premier Daniel Andrews came to national cabinet with an idea that he felt could help address two problems at once. According to an account by *Sydney Morning Herald* journalist Rob Harris, he suggested that all returned travellers should be sent to quarantine in hotels around the country for

14 days. Because Australia had no dedicated quarantine facilities on standby, this was perhaps the only option that could be turned around at speed, to ensure people were isolating properly. 'This is simply a no-brainer,' Andrews reportedly told his fellow leaders.

The decision to require most returning travellers to undertake their mandatory isolation in hotels became the most important decision of Australia's pandemic, setting the country up for its fortuitous but unintended elimination of the virus. But it was a double-edged sword in more ways than one. To begin with, it could not accommodate the number of people who needed it.

Australian Sarah Homewood was sitting on a fluffy rug on the floor of the living room of her apartment in south-east London, crying hysterically. Every fibre of her being was pushing her to pack up her unit, lock the door behind her, and jump on the next plane to Sydney. A public relations manager in her late 20s, she had been living with her husband in a tourist hotspot near London Bridge. As she flicked between the UK and Australian news channels, all of them with wall-to-wall coverage of the global crisis, she listened to prime minister Scott Morrison urging Australians living overseas to return home. But the authorities around the world were also stressing something else: 'Stay put and stay at home.'

It was late March 2020, and London was already in lockdown. Homewood was cautious about taking a seat on a plane from someone who desperately needed it. With the support of their families in Australia, the couple decided to stay on in the UK, where they had built a life with high-flying jobs that they could do from home. But as a grey winter descended, a devastating wave of coronavirus swept through the city, stripping their bustling neighbourhood of all but a few solitary figures. At the supermarkets, terrified Londoners hurried through the aisles. Some wore gas masks, raincoats, and long dishwashing gloves pulled up to their elbows. The pair soon caught the contagion. Homewood lost her sense of smell, and her usually fit-and-healthy husband was pale, slumping breathlessly on a park bench.

When summer came, the warm weather temporarily subdued Covid in Europe. Homewood fell pregnant with her first child, Arthur, in September. It was their plan to return home to Australia for the birth and to be close to their family, but as autumn arrived, another deadly wave of disease hit the UK. The number of quarantine spots available in Australia for returning citizens kept decreasing as Covid kept escaping from quarantine hotels. Homewood found that getting back into the country was not just a lottery, but a lottery that not everyone could buy a ticket in. The only way to secure a seat on a flight out of London was to buy a business-class flight, booked months in advance, she said. Two one-way tickets cost about $30,000, maxing out their credit cards. Every day, they heard stories of other people stranded abroad: people with cancer, and those with nowhere to live because their flights had been cancelled.

Still, many Australians seemed to have little compassion to spare for the stranded citizens, who by September 2020 numbered about 25,000. 'You made a decision to stay, and now you need to live with it,' someone told Homewood, after she wrote about her story in January 2021. 'You are a risk to the rest of the country, and I fully support the way in which the government has managed the cap on arrivals,' commented another. It was strange to be fighting so hard to get home, but also feeling like you were not wanted there.

In her second trimester of pregnancy, she started emailing politicians about her plight, and it was through Tim Wilson, then a government MP in Melbourne, that the couple were suddenly offered a ticket on a flight to Darwin arranged by the Australian government. They had two days to pack up their life in London. The flights and quarantine cost about $10,000. After she boarded the plane at Heathrow Airport on 15 January, Homewood looked around the aisles and saw many other pregnant women, clutching the yellow biosecurity bags with their carry-on belongings, and she felt relieved for them all.

The other major flaw in Australia's hotel quarantine system was that it was regularly failing. The virus is suspected to have escaped more than 30 times in 2020 and 2021, resulting in ten lockdowns spanning six states. High-rise hotels are poor places for infection control, with cramped, windowless corridors and ventilation that pushes the air from guests' rooms out into shared spaces. Dr Omar Khorshid, the president of the Australian Medical Association at the time, said that when considered as a temporary measure, Australia's hotel quarantine system was generally successful and well run. However, as the months ticked by, it became increasingly clear that hotels were not suitable places to keep humans holed up for weeks on end, and that regular breaches were inevitable.

One of the unique things about Australia when it had little or no coronavirus in the community was that every quarantine outbreak was examined in minute detail, and these investigations showed just how hard it was to prevent the virus from escaping. One day in South Australia, an infected guest at the Playford Hotel opened his door to pick up his meal, leaving in the corridor a cloud of virus particles. They were probably still lingering in the air when, 18 seconds later, another guest opened his door. That man would make his way to the outer-Melbourne suburb of Wollert, where the virus would continue its journey, causing another outbreak and another lockdown in Victoria.

The one jurisdiction that didn't see these types of outbreaks was the Northern Territory, and the reason for that seems fairly clear. The territory wasn't housing its arrivals in tourist hotels in cities, but at a disused workers' camp called Howard Springs, just out of Darwin, where cabins with verandas were spaced out in rows. The facility processed more than 64,000 people during the pandemic without a single infection breach.

At one point, the states that relied on hotel quarantine were reporting a virus escaping at a rate of once every 204 infected travellers. The inherent vulnerability of hotels was also magnified by the failure of federal authorities and some jurisdictions to properly recognise the scale of the risk posed by airborne transmission of the virus within hotels. In January 2021, Perth and surrounding suburbs went into a five-day lockdown when a hotel security guard, who had been stationed three metres from the room of an infected guest, but was not wearing a mask of any sort, tested positive. Local officials seemed bamboozled by how it could have happened. 'This is not typical by any means. We know that viruses, such as this, in all but extreme circumstances, transmit from droplets,' a senior health bureaucrat said.

Revered Polish Australian physicist Lidia Morawska knew as soon as she heard Covid-19 was a respiratory virus that it was going to spread through the air. To the scientist, it was an uncontroversial fact that respiratory diseases were, to varying degrees, airborne. However, with the public hungry to understand how they might protect themselves, the World Health Organisation (WHO) was insisting that the virus couldn't travel far because it was mainly spread through large droplets generated when a person coughed, sneezed, or spoke—an assumption grounded in outdated infection-control teachings. This meant people would be able to protect themselves by keeping one metre away from others, disinfecting surfaces frequently, washing their hands, and avoiding touching their eyes, the WHO advised.

It was the last Saturday in March 2020 when Morawska was contacted by a colleague in Italy, engineering professor Giorgio Buonanno. He had a pile of correspondence from local doctors very concerned about the mounting number of Italian healthcare workers dying of Covid-19. 'He was saying, those people are doing everything in the book [to protect themselves], but what wasn't in the book was precaution against airborne transmission.' Many of the nurses and doctors were wearing only a surgical mask or no mask at all, Morawska said, instead of a respirator that would usually be worn for airborne pathogens. It was the same day the WHO had posted an infamous tweet declaring: 'FACT: #Covid19 is NOT airborne.' Buonanno was suggesting the pair petition the Italian authorities about their concerns, but Morawska, who could already see their letter being thrown in the bin by dismissive officials, felt they should aim higher. 'It occurred to me that really we should go after the WHO, because it was the WHO spreading the misinformation.'

Within three days, Morawska had assembled a group of 36 experts on airborne transmission and had fired off an email to senior WHO officials. On 1 April, she was logging on to Zoom and presenting her case to the group of researchers and doctors that advise the WHO on infection containment, armed with evidence that people had been infected with coronavirus even while standing more than a metre away from a contagious person. But Morawska, who had contributed to all of the WHO's air quality guidelines since 1990, felt like she wasn't being taken seriously. 'I didn't have a feeling that they were trying to see this from our perspective,' she said.

Morawska, who lives in Brisbane, would be named one of *Time Magazine*'s most influential people of 2021 for her advocacy, but it would take the WHO another 13 months following this meeting to clearly state that Covid-19 was airborne, and even longer for Australia's federal guidelines to be updated. The delay was perplexing, because Australian researchers produced compelling evidence suggesting that Covid was airborne. Given there was often so little virus in the community—sometimes just one of two cases in the whole country—outbreaks could be meticulously examined. Covid was found to have hopped across hotel corridors, and to have swirled around restaurants.

In July 2020, at least a dozen parishioners caught Covid from an infected musician at a church called the Our Lady of Lebanon in Harris Park, Sydney. The young man had been sitting on an elevated platform 15 metres away from the group (which was equivalent to having a truck between them). He denied touching any objects in the church or mixing with the general congregation, a claim backed by video of the service. Associate Professor Stephen Corbett, who was involved in investigating the outbreak with the public health unit in Western Sydney, said the cone-shaped design of the cathedral was key, as it caused air to be pushed up, run along a wall, waft past the choral chamber where the musician was sitting, and then tip over into the congregation.

In January the next year, Corbett also helped investigate an outbreak at a Berala bottle shop in Sydney where CCTV captured the moment it was suspected a patron caught Covid from another customer. The pair were no closer than five metres. Corbett, a senior public health doctor with four decades' experience, said before the Covid pandemic began, he was already aware from Lidia Morawska's 'groundbreaking research' that coronaviruses could spread over longer distances. He believes the resistance to acknowledging airborne transmission of the new virus was partly driven by the massive implications that acknowledgement had for infection control.

'The prospect that airborne infection is a serious issue in health-care settings is daunting, because it means people have to be swaddled up in uncomfortable clothing to do their everyday work.'

In March and April 2020, stories poured in from Australian nurses and healthcare workers who said they were being denied access to masks, amid a global shortage of protective equipment. Some were even told they couldn't bring in their own from home. A junior doctor working at a Covid clinic was instructed that they didn't need any protective gear unless they were performing a physical exam of a patient. A paramedic said that the ambulance service they worked for told them, 'as per WHO recommendations', a splash gown was all that was needed to treat Covid-19 patients. General practitioners resorted to buying goggles from hardware shops as makeshift eye protection. There were hundreds of stories like this.

Professor Julian Rait, the Victorian president of the Australian Medical Association, said the 'biggest stuff-up of the entire pandemic' was the reluctance of governments to accept the threat of airborne spread early on. 'They were just sticking to the old dogma,' Rait said. The ophthalmologist was one of the first health experts in the country to push for properly fitted N95 respirators to be mandated in hospitals to protect frontline workers from airborne spread. When the first Australian healthcare worker was hospitalised with the virus in early 2020 in New South Wales, Rait said he became very concerned. His daughter, Louise, was working as a junior doctor at the Royal Melbourne Hospital. In

2020, more than 3,000 Victorian healthcare workers were infected with the virus.

Investigators would later find it was common for air in rooms of sick patients to be funnelled into busy corridors, with poor ventilation and airflow problems the root cause of many coronavirus outbreaks in hospitals. Delirious aged-care patients shouting and roaming in hospital wards expelling virus particles in the air were also linked to virus super-spreading events.

Scott Morrison said he had a conversation with UK prime minister Boris Johnson very early on in the pandemic about whether it might be possible to let the virus come into the country and then manage it. Coronavirus deaths in the UK would reach more than 1,300 a day by early April 2020, and the British government, which briefly flirted with the controversial concept of 'herd immunity', would be accused of taking a fatalistic approach to letting the virus spread. Morrison believes it was an exaggeration that the UK was pursuing a herd immunity approach: a strategy whereby authorities deliberately allow a large proportion of their population to get infected, hoping it will build up immunity to the virus. In any case, he said this sort of approach was never contemplated in Australia. The advice Morrison was receiving was that it wasn't clear if infection with coronavirus caused lasting immunity, and there was still significant uncertainty about what harm the virus would be exposing the population to.

'The fact that there was no vaccine, and we had no idea how bad this was going to be at that point, meant that we just couldn't take that risk,' he said. 'I mean, we weren't so naive to think that it wouldn't come and it wouldn't have its impact, but we knew we could slow it down. That's what we knew we could do. We could flatten the curve.'

What might surprise many Australians, and rankle others, is that sweeping lockdowns and international border closures were never part of the plan. According to the Australian Health Management Plan for Pandemic Influenza, there were several measures that authorities could call on in the inevitable scenario that the nation was faced with a new pandemic. Social distancing was among them, but school closures, workplace shutdowns, and bans on mass gatherings were generally not recommended, unless the pandemic was at the more serious end of the scale. The plan certainly didn't envisage a scenario in which people were only allowed to leave their homes for a small number of essential reasons, nor did it foresee anything close to a monitored 14-day quarantine.

Professor James McCaw, who helped develop the pandemic plan, said that if anyone had asked him prior to Covid-19 if forcing people to stay in an organised quarantine facility for two virus incubation periods would stop the disease getting in the country, his answer would have been 'Yes.' But this measure wasn't written into the plan, because it was thought it wouldn't be accepted by the community, and therefore not palatable for politicians. It was the same with lockdowns. 'Anyone who works in my area could have told you if you shut down a society, you will stop the virus, [but] there is no pandemic plan that I know of anywhere in the world that recommended lockdowns,' McCaw said. He said he 'would have been laughed out of the room' if he had tried to suggest it.

Victoria's chief health officer, Brett Sutton, told us that officials and experts were prompted to rethink their assumptions as they looked beyond Australia and saw hospital systems straining under coronavirus cases and the rationing of intensive-care beds in Italy's Lombardy region. Millions of Italians were locked down in early March. Then there was China, which by the end of February was beginning to drive cases down through lockdowns. That suggested it might be possible to gain some control over the virus. Sutton said officials around the globe moved from the assumption that the Western world could never contemplate the idea of a lockdown to believing it might be the thing required to address the extraordinary challenge they were facing.

'I think Italy demonstrated that (a) it was necessary, and (b) it was something that the population was prepared to go to as a measure to deal with what was an overwhelming situation,' he said.

The purpose of the initial border closure and national lockdown had been to slow the spread of coronavirus, to give the hospitals time to prepare and stagger the wave of illness.

'We needed to buy ourselves some time to learn more about the disease, and what the true implications of it were [and to] build up our medical resources,' said Steven Marshall, the South Australian premier. It was not expected that these steps would temporarily eliminate the disease from the community. Several leading public health experts say the initial success of these radical measures left them grappling with a strange if not welcome quandary. What now?

CHAPTER SEVEN

Tasmania's moat

Many ships have been lost in the Bass Strait, the dangerous stretch of ocean that separates the Australian mainland from the island state of Tasmania. Before improvements in marine navigation, vessels were regularly battered and broken in its waters.

Peter Gutwein, who was elected as Tasmania's 46th premier as the Covid pandemic began, said that for two centuries the island state's single largest ailment was its geographical position, as an isolated island at the bottom of the continent. 'We struggled with the tyranny of distance,' he said. But for a period of time, the 250 kilometres of inhospitable sea between Victoria and its southern neighbour became its 'greatest strength', Gutwein said.

On 19 March 2020, Tasmania was the first state to announce an effective closing of its domestic borders, in defiance of the wishes of prime minister Scott Morrison. From the next day, all but a select group of essential visitors, such as truck drivers and defence force personnel, had to quarantine for 14 days on arrival. Tasmania's tourism and hospitality industries were crippled, although many businesses big and small were already making the decision to shut their doors ahead of any formal directions.

Hobart's most famous attraction, the Museum of Old and New Art, nicknamed Mona, had announced its closure to visitors two days earlier. Owner David Walsh, who had built his fortune as a professional gambler, said he agonised over whether keeping the museum open would benefit or harm the community, but had eventually settled on the precautionary principle. 'Mona, most likely, would play no part in the spread of this insidious coronavirus, and so closing would, probably, play no part in protecting against it,' he wrote. 'But there's a chance that Mona could become a major centre for contagion.'

Gutwein believed that the Australian federation of states provided Tasmania with a model for how it might manage things. 'I use the analogy of a ship with watertight compartments. If there is a problem with one compartment, you close it off. In our case, the federation drew lines on the map, and we were at liberty to make decisions in terms of our own state borders,' he told us. 'It was determined that the best and safest route for Tasmania was, as an island, to close its borders at that time.'

While the prime minister may not have been a fan of the decision, the front page of Hobart's daily newspaper, *The Mercury*, the following morning gave a strong indication of where local sentiment lay. Set against a map of Tasmania, with a gloomy dark-blue ocean around it, was the headline: 'We've got a moat, and we're not afraid to use it.' The paper praised the premier for his 'gutsy call', which had the backing of the state's Labor opposition and the Greens.

To restrict arrivals at the border, a state of emergency was declared, and the state's police commissioner, Darren Hine, was installed as state controller. He was joined by Tasmania's health department secretary, Kathrine Morgan-Wicks, and the director of public health, Dr Mark Veitch, in the premier's core team of pandemic advisers and decision-makers. The officials were motivated by a well-founded fear that the island could run out of ventilators, and that its 41 intensive-care beds would be quickly overrun.

Tasmania has the oldest population in the nation, with more than 20 per cent of residents aged 65 or older, and a small and often stressed health system. Dr Veitch said domestic visitor restrictions were considered particularly advantageous in Tasmania because the state didn't have a busy international airport, and cruise ships were banned from docking in Tasmania from mid-March 2020. 'So we actually had a reasonable likelihood of not importing too many cases directly the way other jurisdictions would with international arrivals,' the chief public health official said.

Kathrine Morgan-Wicks, a lawyer by trade who had previously led the state's justice department, had been transferred to lead the Tasmanian health department in September 2019, and had been tasked with sorting out budget deficits. Instead, the pandemic ushered in new priorities, and she found herself being told by the premier, 'Kath, spend what you need to—just do it.' As officials scrambled to secure important supplies, the bureaucrat sat in an emergency control centre in April 2020 being handed one paper contract after another. In a single day, she estimates she signed for roughly $40 million worth of purchases. She leased a helicopter. Forty thousand litres of alcohol-based hand sanitiser were ordered from local whisky and gin distilleries, which had pivoted their production to the pandemic efforts.

Officials were working until 1.00 am or 2.00 am, day after day, spending countless hours trying to source N95 masks and ventilators. Morgan-Wicks said it left them feeling like arms traffickers. 'We'd get these calls and emails from all over the world saying, "We're on the tarmac somewhere in the Philippines with 100 ventilators—do you want them?"'

Hours before Tasmania's border was closed on 20 March 2020, a group of 54 holiday-makers had slipped back into the state, having just disembarked from the Ruby Princess cruise liner in Sydney. Although they didn't yet know it, 18 of them had coronavirus. Three of the infected travellers were hospitalised at the North West Regional Hospital, a 160-bed facility in the small port town of Burnie. By early the next month, the disease had spread from two of the returned passengers to staff at the hospital, triggering a rolling outbreak among workers and patients that progressively paralysed the hospital. Medical and surgical wards were closed, and the facility was shut off to visitors.

Then a change was made to the national definition of close contacts that drastically increased the number of workers forced into isolation. Previously, people were only deemed close contacts if they had spent at least 15 minutes continuously with someone who had tested positive for coronavirus. After the new definition, it didn't matter if the 15 minutes had been in short stints, or not. 'With that definition change, it changed everything,' said Morgan-Wicks, who had earlier established an incident-management team for the unfolding emergency. 'We had to put entire wards into closure, and by Easter Thursday and then Good Friday, we were running out of people to man the hospital.' The staff shortages were so dire that the hospital's general manager was helping at the mortuary, because there was no one else left to prepare the deceased. By Easter Saturday, a call was made to shut down the entire facility by Monday, as well as the neighbouring private hospital. Every single person who had worked at the two hospitals and related medical services since 27 March, as well as their household members, went into quarantine for 14 days.

This meant that almost 5,000 people were in isolation, equivalent to a quarter of the population of Burnie. In the surrounding area, stricter social-distancing restrictions were ushered in, forcing the closure of schools and all non-essential businesses, including the department stores Target and Kmart. Closing the two hospitals was the hardest decision of Morgan-Wicks' life, because she knew it meant shutting off the entire north-west corner of Tasmania to emergency health care. She said local authorities initially 'really had to beg' the federal health department for assistance from the defence force to keep basic urgent medical support available.

The premier had left Hobart on Thursday that week to try to snatch a few days over Easter with his wife and two teenage children, but was back in the state capital by Saturday as the situation escalated. As became his practice through the pandemic, Gutwein walked alone for hours through the streets of Hobart's CBD. He was mulling over the enormity of what he was going to announce the next day: the closure of two hospitals on Easter Sunday. He spoke to the prime minister, who he said told him the Commonwealth would provide the Tasmanian government with 'whatever support you need'. But even the physical act of closing the hospitals wasn't as simple as it sounds. There were no locks on the front doors, because hospitals usually operate 24 hours a day, seven days a week.

Likewise, some of the equipment had never been switched off before. The incident management team had to contact nearly every cleaning company in the state to cobble together a crew to scour the two hospitals. The group included out-of-work cleaners from the Spirit of Tasmania ferry, and staff from mum-and-dad cleaning businesses, who were given two days' training in wearing protective gear before venturing into the empty buildings in full-body gowns, removing blood and vomit bags from the abandoned emergency department. 'These people were heroes in my opinion—everyone was frightened to enter the hospital,' Morgan-Wicks said.

All the heavily pregnant women due to give birth in Burnie, now marooned from care, were called, and were set up in accommodation in Launceston, almost two hours away. And in an extraordinary deployment, the Australian defence force sent doctors, emergency nurses, a pharmacist, and a radiographer among a team of 50 people to reopen the emergency department at the North West Regional Hospital, restoring basic urgent care for the weeks that the regular staff were quarantined. They were joined by seven people from the Australian Medical Assistance Teams—the same service that had been sent to repatriate passengers from the Diamond Princess.

The Burnie disaster is the best local example of what would have played out nationally in the early months of 2020 if the nation's borders hadn't been closed and Australians had not embraced social-distancing measures. Commonwealth chief medical officer Paul Kelly told us that Australia was no different from the rest of the world in that respect. It would have been 'Burnie on a scale that you cannot imagine', he said, if Covid-19 had been allowed to spread through the country, through one unvaccinated community after the next. 'We would have run out of staff. We would not have had enough ventilators. We would not have had enough trained people,' Kelly said. 'We do have a strong health system, we have universal insurance coverage through Medicare, we have extremely well-trained staff, but even the best of systems broke during this time, and we would have been the same.'

At least ten people, most of them hospital patients in their 70s, 80s, and 90s, died in the Burnie cluster, and dozens of healthcare staff developed long Covid, post-traumatic stress disorder, or other persistent symptoms. Morgan-Wicks said the state learnt 'hard and fast' that to have a functioning health system they needed to pour everything they had into protecting the island and its old and vulnerable population, until vaccinations arrived. 'We couldn't burn like that,' she said. 'We couldn't burn like we did in the north-west and survive this.'

No one alive had dealt with a pandemic on the scale the world was encountering, and Gutwein is very conscious that his experience as premier, a role he began in January 2020, was far removed from that of his recent predecessors. For two years, he remained largely domiciled in the south of the state, away from his family in the north and his home in Launceston.

Looking back, he said the difficult decisions he and his advisers had to take, based on what they considered to be the best available information, bordered on the surreal. The sweeping shutdown of the state, echoed across the nation in late March, temporarily closed hotels, museums, gyms, community centres, markets, churches, and swimming pools. 'All of my life I've worked to create things and build things, and have been involved in small to medium enterprises, and I understood how difficult it would be for those businesses we closed,' said Gutwein, a former treasurer. 'To say that we wrestled with these matters would be an understatement.'

Gutwein recalls putting 'helicopters in the sky' and setting up police roadblocks during Easter 2020 as authorities ordered people not to holiday at their coastal properties, worried they would spread coronavirus into communities of retirees. Soon after the border restrictions were introduced, his staff began forwarding him emails from Tasmanians distressed that their family and friends interstate were barred from attending funerals in Tasmania. Among the cases was a family that had lost their teenage son. The boy's brother had been due to fly home to Tasmania for the funeral. Gutwein said he spoke to the police commissioner about how they might accommodate something like this, and the police chief had told him, 'Look, we don't.' The commissioner offered to make the call to the family, but Gutwein felt a responsibility to break the news to them himself. 'Obviously, they were devastated … It was relayed to me that his mother felt that she was losing her second son, because he couldn't come home for the funeral.' Several years later, Gutwein said he did not regret the decision. Similar gatherings interstate had proven to be catalysts for the coronavirus spreading. '[It] greatly distressed me at the time, but I knew that to do otherwise would risk other Tasmanian lives."

In the midst of this all, there was an election. Gutwein was returned to office in May 2021. It was an unprecedented result for the Tasmanian Liberal Party, the first time it had won three consecutive elections. Observers said the government's successful handling of Covid was a key factor in the victory. After the initial shock of the autumn 2020 lockdown, the Tasmanian economy was growing at twice the national average. Even interstate travellers were welcomed back, provided they were from states that had similarly controlled the virus. But Gutwein was burning out. A few days before he was due to take leave during the July 2021 school holidays, he was woken at 3.00 am by a ping on his mobile phone. It was an email from a Victorian teacher telling him that a schoolgirl visiting Tasmania for a chess championship was now a Covid-19 close contact, and that she had been at about 25 to 30 different places in the state in the preceding 24 hours. That an ordinary member of the public was able to directly email a premier, rousing him in the middle of the night, may seem bizarre to outsiders, but it says a lot about the public's access to politicians in Australia's smallest state.

In fact, when we sought to interview Gutwein about Tasmania's pandemic experience, we were surprised to receive a direct message from him on WhatsApp, not long after we had called a former adviser asking him if he might be prepared to chat. Other meetings with pandemic premiers and chief health officers had taken many weeks or months to secure, and numerous back-and-forths with their minders, seeking a list of potential questions. It was a blustery day when we flew into Launceston to meet the high-profile Tasmanian. Gutwein met us at a CBD café, pulling a beanie off his shaven head as he walked through the door. He greeted a table of diners, and perhaps there was a quiet glance from the other customers, but his presence otherwise went politely unremarked.

The alert involving the Victorian school students ended up being a false alarm of sorts. The group were placed in isolation, where they all tested negative for Covid. However, by then an outbreak that had begun in Sydney was threatening to take hold in Melbourne, and there was never time for Gutwein to take a holiday. The premier had worked for 46 days without a break, when in late August he woke up feeling not quite himself. As was his custom, he made his way into his Hobart office, starting work at around 7.15 am.

'At nine o'clock, I thought I'll go and get a coffee, and have a walk and smarten myself up a bit with some fresh air. I had a quick walk around a couple of blocks and went back to the office, and didn't feel much better—in fact, I started to feel a little worse,' Gutwein recalled. 'I then thought, for some odd reason, that I needed to find the coldest place in the building and get some air there. So I caught a lift down to the second floor, which is a car park … walked out of the lift, and fell over on my backside.'

News quickly broke that the premier had collapsed at work, but hospital doctors could find no sinister underlying illness in the 56-year-old. The episode had been caused by overwork. The prescribed treatment was to take a couple of days off, sitting on the couch at home in Launceston watching television, and to try not to think about work too much. The medieval drama *Game of Thrones* was his show of choice.

Tasmania came very close to being the only state in Australia to avoid any further lockdowns after the first wave of disease, in an unbroken stint that lasted about 15 months. Then came along a bloke called Timothy Andrew Gunn. There were plenty of people during the pandemic who unwittingly became public enemies because of small, regrettable mistakes. Gunn does not fall into that category. The 31-year-old from Albury-Wodonga gained entry to Tasmania illegally by lying about where he lived. Flying in on the evening Jetstar flight on 11 October 2021, he had already had two recent entry applications rejected because he had been living in a Covid hotspot.

Upon his arrival, Gunn was moved into a quarantine hotel at Hobart's Travelodge, where it is thought that he slipped out of a fire escape while security guards briefly left their posts to change their protective clothing. It took over 12 hours before it was confirmed that he was missing, after several calls to his room had gone unanswered. The escapee was discovered by police at a garage in the suburb of Bridgewater late the next afternoon, by which point he had visited a supermarket while, it turns out, he was positive to a strain of Covid.

Gutwein told parliament a couple of days later that Gunn had been refusing to wear a mask since his apprehension and was 'not being cooperative, and in fact has been very difficult to deal with'. Because officials felt they could not trust the information they were receiving from him, it was decided to enforce 'a short, sharp lockdown' of Hobart and southern Tasmania lasting three days, by which time they established that the disease hadn't jumped into the community. 'We don't want to be Sydney or Melbourne … that acted too late,' Gutwein said at the time. The public were only allowed to move within five kilometres of their home to go shopping for essentials, and two hours every day to exercise. Gunn, dubbed 'possibly the most hated man in Tasmania', later claimed in an interview with Seven News that he didn't think he had to stay at hotel quarantine, and he hoped that Tasmanians would find it in their hearts to forgive him.

The pandemic led to a rapid change in the way many people in affluent countries lived and worked. The number of Australians reporting working from home at least one day a week doubled to 40 per cent within a few months in 2020. Many office employees were happy to ditch their commute as often as they could, even after lock-downs were lifted. It was no longer possible for many employers to say that working from home wasn't feasible. Some people went a step further, moving not just out of CBD offices, but out of major cities entirely, in search of an ocean or a forest, having spent too long restricted to the same dreary suburban streets and local parks. Burnout became another buzzword, mostly among healthcare workers facing record numbers of sick patients without any respite, but also among parents having to juggle remote schooling, and others at the frontline of the pandemic.

In March 2022, Gutwein was sitting around the breakfast table at his home in Launceston for a fifth day in a row. He was only there and not in Hobart because his teenage daughter Millie had tested positive for Covid, and the family were observing the isolation period. 'Today's a day for celebration,' declared his wife, Amanda. 'Five days under this roof is the longest you've spent in this house in nearly two years.' By that evening, Gutwein had resolved to quit politics. It was like an epiphany, he said.

Initially, his chief-of-staff, Andrew Finch, talked him into staying until July or August, in order to deliver the budget and other big-ticket items. But a few days later he was in the middle of a press conference with prime minister Scott Morrison, talking about a proposed elec-tricity and telecommunications link between Tasmania and Victoria, when he was again hit by the feeling he didn't want to spend a second longer living away from his family.

Many were shocked when he announced his retirement the next day. In the cut-throat world of Australian politics, most premiers and prime ministers find themselves voted, or otherwise forced, out of their job. Few leave on their own terms, at least before the pandemic. Although he spent just two years as premier, it followed eight years as the state's treasurer, and capped off two decades in parliament. He was, he said, satisfied after 'guiding Tasmanians through a particularly tough period'.

Gutwin often declared in speeches that Tasmania was 'one of the safest places on the planet'. After the Burnie outbreak, not a single person died of Covid until more than 90 per cent of the state's eligible population had been doubly vaccinated and the government chose to open up to Covid-19, almost two years later. 'I've focused on everyone else's family, I now want to spend some time focusing on my own,' Gutwein said. 'What I've found after the last two years especially is I have nothing left in the tank to give.'

CHAPTER EIGHT

A hidden wave

Late one evening in June 2020, a young scientist named Courtney Lane was staring in shock at the laptop in front of her. Sitting on her couch in her track pants in her art-deco apartment in Melbourne's north, she had made an explosive discovery. Displayed on the screen, in a mess of dots and lines, was the genomic data of the cases in the new outbreak that had emerged in Melbourne. They could be traced back, almost entirely, to a breach from a hotel that the government had been using to quarantine Covid-positive returned travellers from overseas.

'I remember opening up the phylogenetic tree, and having a look and overlaying the epidemiological data and just having that moment of like, *Oh, God, it's very very very clear what has happened here,*' said Lane, an infectious disease epidemiologist at the Doherty Institute. The data showed that coronavirus had made its way from a family that had flown in from Bangladesh on 9 May and been quarantined at the Rydges hotel in Melbourne's CBD for two weeks. Within weeks, a hotel staff member and two security guards had developed symptoms of the virus. One of the infected guards remembers feeling feverish during a shift in late May, looking around and noticing that other hotel workers were sniffling. Thinking he had a cold, he spent the next three days travelling across Melbourne working as a food-delivery driver. By the time of Lane's discovery about a month later, more than 300 Victorians had been infected with Covid-19.

Dr Norelle Sherry, a clinical microbiologist at the Doherty Institute, remembers that it was about 9.00 pm or 10.00 pm when Lane called and told her, 'I think the second wave has come from hotel quarantine ... Can you please check? Because we really need to be 100 per cent sure about this.' What Sherry observed in the data was very different from the first wave in Victoria, when more than 30 separate introductions of coronavirus from returned travellers around March each resulted in just a handful of cases before petering out. But the second-wave cases Lane was examining had remarkably similar genomics, meaning they were connected, and they certainly weren't fading away.

Lane and Sherry called their boss, Professor Ben Howden, the director of the Microbiological Diagnostic Unit Public Health Laboratory. It was his job to relay the findings to senior management at the Victorian health department. Howden said they were pretty shocked to hear the news. 'In another country where they weren't trying to completely stop importation, it wouldn't have been such a big deal, but in our country it was a very big deal.'

The next day, a grim-faced Daniel Andrews walked into the theatrette at Melbourne's Treasury Place, dressed in a navy-blue blazer and checked cream shirt. The premier did what journalists call 'burying the lede'. This is when the most important elements of a story are buried deep down below details and distracting information.

In front of socially distanced television crews and journalists scattered across rows of seats in a vast theatre, he revealed that the Doherty's genomic testing had indicated that a number of Victorian cases in late May and early June could be linked to a breach of the hotel quarantine program. Retired judge Jennifer Coate had already been appointed to lead an inquiry into the operation of the program, he told the public.

'Clearly, there has been a failure, 'Andrews said. The premier then swiftly turned the blame on the security guards and staff, who he said had broken 'well-known and well understood infection-control protocols'. 'That is unacceptable to me,' he said. 'I'm sure that it will be unacceptable certainly to all of those who will be impacted by the restrictions that we have had to reimpose.'

The bombshell news that Victoria's new coronavirus wave had come from a government-operated quarantine hotel would normally have been seized by the media and would have dominated their reports, but it was completely trumped by what came next. Standing in front of a giant purple banner with state government branding and emblazoned with the words 'Staying apart keeps us together', Andrews announced a drastic reimposition of coronavirus restrictions.

The state had just recorded 64 new coronavirus infections, and ten postcodes—taking in 36 suburbs in Melbourne's north and north-west, considered virus hotspots—were being sent into lockdown from midnight. The premier read out the postcodes and suburbs one by one: 3012: Brooklyn, Kingsville, Maidstone, Tottenham, West Footscray; 3021: Albanvale, Kealba, Kings Park, St Albans; 3032: Ascot Vale, Highpoint City, Maribyrnong, Travancore; and on it went.

The only reason people could leave their home was to exercise, work, buy essential items such as food and medicine, or access childcare and health care. International flights coming into Melbourne were to be diverted. As more than 1,000 police were deployed into the hotspots, the new rules came with a warning from Andrews that Victoria Police will 'not be mucking about'. Drones circled public spaces, tracking the movements of about 300,000 Melburnians. A booze-bus style police operation was enforced, and policing units used number-plate recognition to scan drivers' cars. Those trying to leave or enter the suburbs were questioned by police, and residents were ordered to carry their driver's licence with their current address.

While the government scrambled to contain the virus in the ten postcodes, there was more anxious chatter among senior government and public health officials about another potentially looming disaster. Rising coronavirus infections were being detected in several of Melbourne's public housing towers. Overcrowding and shared facilities meant that the outbreak had the potential to take off. Then, on 4 July 2020, something unimaginable happened.

The blinding blue-and-red lights came suddenly, bathing the austere concrete walls of the towering Flemington housing estate late on that wintry afternoon, as Victorian premier Daniel Andrews' press conference was broadcast to televisions in living rooms across the state. Hundreds of police swarmed the high-rise flats. The residents thought there had been a mass shooting, a murder, or a terrorism attack. They scrambled down the stairs, spilling out of rickety lifts onto the ground floor. Wide-eyed children clutched their parents, confused and frightened. 'Why are the police coming here?' they asked. 'Are they coming here to catch criminals?'

By 4.00 pm that day, nine high-rise public housing towers in Melbourne—home to more than 3,000 people from the state's most culturally diverse, poor, and at-risk communities—were placed into a hard lockdown under police guard with no warning.

The snap lockdown made global headlines. Built as part of the post-World War II slum-clearance project, the flats were a towering presence on the skyline of the now-gentrified inner-city suburbs of North Melbourne and Flemington. People who returned home that night as the sky darkened, without identification to prove they lived in the flats, were turned away and locked out of their own homes. It became evident the state government had locked down the towers without planning ahead for how it was going to provide the most basic necessities to the residents inside, who hailed from about 80 countries and spoke more than 30 languages.

Nor Shanino was raised in the flats on Racecourse Road in Flemington, and worked as a community volunteer during the lockdown, helping those locked inside the towers, including his sister, father, and stepmother. Days after the lockdown began, Shanino witnessed a frail, elderly African woman with hollow eyes and sunken cheeks shivering as she staggered into the North Melbourne mosque. It is a sight he will never forget. Not long before, the woman had moved into the flats after fleeing an abusive relationship. Shanino said she barely spoke a word of English and had been left stranded after arriving without any identification to prove where she lived. For days, she slept rough in bitterly cold conditions in a broken-down car parked outside the flats. 'She had a heart condition and a whole bunch of other health issues,' said Shanino, who lived in nearby North Melbourne. 'By the time we saw her, she could barely speak. We sat her down and got her some water before a couple of volunteers took her to the hospital. They discovered she had hypothermia.'

There were so many stories like this, Shanino said. 'There was an assumption, deeply rooted in racism, that everyone in the towers would run away, they would try and escape, they needed to be locked up, under police guard, like a prison,' he said. 'That for whatever reason they did not deserve the respect of having time to stock up on medicine and food that was granted to every other Australian who was put into a lockdown.'

Police surrounded the public housing towers, guarding the entrances to the flats and setting up checkpoints, which blocked off deliveries of food and urgent medicine. Families in precarious financial situations, whose weekly ritual is to often shop for their groceries on Sunday afternoons, were left with little or no food. Victorian ombudsman Deborah Glass, who investigated the lockdown, was told that some residents could hear their neighbours screaming as their mental health deteriorated, their howls echoing down the empty hallways of the high-rise flats.

The strict quarantine lasted five days for most, but two weeks for people living in the North Melbourne public housing flats. Youth worker Barry Berih was inside his flat in the North Melbourne towers on Alfred Street when Andrews announced the lockdown. Berih grabbed his phone and began calling his neighbours. He hastily created WhatsApp and Facebook groups to circulate information about the outbreak and to provide support for residents. His overwhelming concern was for his elderly neighbours, many of who spoke no English and had serious underlying medical conditions.

One of Berih's neighbours, a father-of-two in his 70s, died after being infected with the virus during the lockdown. Berih had known the man most of his life, often praying at the local mosque with him. 'His family is still coming to terms with it,' said Berih, 27, who was born in Australia to Eritrean parents. Berih said the haphazard way the lockdown was enforced meant there were initial delays in paramedics and doctors being able to get inside the flats to treat the ill, like his neighbour who died.

'The ambulances were parked downstairs, but some residents were waiting hours when they needed urgent medical help,' he said.

Berih and his younger brother both caught Covid during the outbreak as they ran between flats, dropping off food and medicine left in bags outside the towers by volunteers. Their mother, Kubra, was locked out of the flats after returning home from a shift as a hospital cleaner without identification to prove she lived there. She spent the next week staying with relatives a few suburbs away. Like many living in the towers, Berih said the lockdown left him questioning his identity as an Australian. 'Why were we treated so differently to everybody else? You feel like a second-class citizen. Like you're not an Australian after all.'

Politicians and health department leaders who had made the call to go against expert health advice and to push the lockdown forward by 36 hours in a secret crisis cabinet meeting were nowhere to be seen when community legal worker Anthony Kelly arrived at the Flemington towers hours after the lockdown was announced. 'I just remember I kept asking, "Who is in charge here?"' Kelly, who was head of the Flemington Legal Community Centre, said. 'Nobody knew. It was shockingly incompetent. There was just no line of command. No leadership. No accountability from the government.'

By all accounts, Dr Annaliese van Diemen, a young public health physician, who at the time was acting for Brett Sutton as Victoria's chief health officer, was ambushed. She was left with just minutes to weigh up the complexities of the human rights implications of this lockdown of thousands of Victorians.

An email landed in van Diemen's inbox just 15 minutes before a press conference on 4 July. It detailed the proposed directions of the public housing lockdown—in what would become the first use of emergency detention powers in Australia to manage an outbreak of Covid-19.

Van Diemen, who signed off on the directions in Sutton's absence, scrambled to scan the document on her mobile phone in the car on her way to the press conference. She would later describe the uneasiness she felt, telling Glass she would have preferred to have had longer to consider the human rights implications of the lockdown. Perhaps the most troubling part of van Diemen's submission to the ombudsman was that, even if she had wanted to 'put the brakes on the thing', she said she wouldn't have felt comfortable doing so.

Van Dieman was adamant that the immediacy of the lockdown was not part of her advice. Despite being the most senior public health official on the day, she was not even consulted about bringing the lockdown forward. She had assumed it would go ahead 36 hours later, as planned, leaving residents with enough time to gather the supplies they needed. 'I was quite terrified, to be honest, that we would see within a week many hundreds of cases. It was a very, very difficult decision. I absolutely didn't take it lightly,' she told Glass. But, she added, 'I don't think that one day would've made a hugely significant difference to the longer-term epidemiology of that outbreak.' In a telling sign of the personal toll the ordeal took on van Diemen, she asked to be shifted off the pandemic-response team soon after.

Emergency management commissioner Andrew Crisp told the ombudsman that the timing of the intervention 'firmed up' throughout the late morning and early afternoon, but even he couldn't pinpoint who told him it had been brought forward 36 hours from the original plan. When asked by the ombudsman to provide details of what was discussed at that meeting, and why the lockdown had been brought forward, the premier, Daniel Andrews, refused, citing cabinet confidentiality. But in its submission to the ombudsman, the Victorian Department of Health wrote: 'There are people alive today who may not have been alive if the department had not acted so quickly.'

That this outbreak was handled in such a way in a city like Melbourne was appalling, Anthony Kelly said. Certainly, he acknowledged, these were crisis times, and lives were undeniably at stake, but the excessive haste in shutting down the towers meant there was poor logistical preparation, no clear plan to provide necessities, along with inadequate consideration of the human rights implications for residents. 'It was a situation akin to a humanitarian crisis,' said Kelly, whose workplace has for more than a decade provided legal aid to the diverse migrant population residing there. 'The dynamics were very similar to a refugee camp, or a conflict zone, where a large population had been suddenly displaced and was experiencing food and medicine scarcity.' Kelly remembered people sleeping in parked cars out the front of the Flemington estate, and distressed parents begging to be allowed back into the flats where their young or teenage children were. 'One single father couldn't get access to his children, and they couldn't get out,' said Kelly, who was asked by the ombudsman to monitor the situation for the human rights commission. 'He was just completely distraught.'

In the end, it was the Australian Muslim Social Services Agency (AMSSA) and volunteers like Berih and Shanino, who, after coming up against initial resistance from authorities and police, became the heart of the relief effort. They used their local knowledge, language, and, most crucially, the trust they had with the residents to try to mitigate the worst effects of the lockdown. Within hours, a disused warehouse in North Melbourne that AMSSA used as a mosque and community centre was overflowing with thousands of green-and-white shopping bags filled with food donations, face masks, and other essentials. Days later, volunteers in the warehouse were tailoring care packages to residents. But they still faced a struggle with authorities to get medical and food supplies to the residents, with police sporadically intercepting and searching cars on arrival.

Another blow came when, in a response to the volunteers' attempt to organise fresh air and exercise at the Alfred Street towers, authorities erected a wire fence around the entrance. Berih remembers it vividly: 'I looked at it, and I saw this cage. And I thought, *Well, that is it. They really have put us in prison. We are in jail now.*' Years later, it is still called 'the cage' by residents, who thought it resembled a cattle pen used for herding animals. The fence was dismantled quickly after protests from residents and community members. The ombudsman later described it as 'clearly degrading and inhumane'.

Kelly remained frustrated by what he described as an extreme police response at the towers, which seemed to ignore the chief health officer's directive that people should be allowed to leave for health and safety purposes. 'The police either weren't instructed about that, or what they were enforcing was a rigid, no-exemptions lockdown,' Kelly said. 'Residents who had valid reasons to leave their homes, such as to get medical assistance, were being simply given a blanket no.'

While no one argues that decisive government intervention was not necessary to stop the spread of Covid in the public housing towers, the abruptness of the lockdown was deemed a violation of human rights by ombudsman Glass. She noted that the overpowering police presence severely traumatised those living in the towers, many of whom had fled war-torn countries. 'Their distress, when they spoke to us, was palpable,' Glass said. She found that while the lockdown itself was justified on public health grounds, the immediacy of it was not, and the government had assumed the towers were 'a hotbed of criminality and non-compliance. But the evidence was the vast majority were law-abiding people, just like other Australians. It is unimaginable that such stereotypical assumptions, leading to "the theatre of policing" that followed, would have accompanied the response to an outbreak of Covid-19 in a luxury apartment block.'

Nor Shanino remembered tensions boiling over between police and volunteers when a young resident in the grips of a psychotic episode ran out of the towers. As he charged towards the police, volunteers who knew the man stepped in to calm him down, and a tense stand-off occurred with the police. The incident was captured on camera by TV crews. 'We told the cops if something happens with a resident, reach out to us and see if we can resolve it because we know them, and if we can't resolve it, the police can step in,' Shanino said. 'From then on, the police never had to step in again.'

The government had wanted to save lives, and arguably it did. But what eats away at Glass most is the government's complete failure to seek properly considered advice, particularly on the human rights implications of the public health order, which she said rendered this lockdown unlawful. 'There just wasn't a public health justification for pushing the lockdown forward, and that is where the government's argument is fundamentally flawed,' she said during an interview in her second-floor office overlooking Bourke Street in Melbourne's CBD in early 2022. 'In a just society, human rights are not a convention to be ignored during a crisis, but a framework for how we will treat and be treated as the crisis unfolds.' Put simply, Glass said, the lockdown was treated as a security operation, and not as a public health response.

'What got up my nose the most was the way this played out in public commentary. This idea that they had to lock them down because otherwise they would all have escaped and endangered the rest of us,' Glass said. 'Well, hang on a second. Where were these 3,000 residents going to run to? Where were they going to go? Check into a hotel?' Glass said she could not even blame 'Victoria's obsession with Covid zero', because all the other state lockdowns were done with adequate notice.

Ruth Eyakem still remembers the fear she felt as she heard Andrews announce the lockdown on television. She peered outside to see the police gathering below, then raced downstairs, hoping to make it to the chemist in time to fill a prescription for her anxiety medication that had just run out. But when she tried to leave the building, the police told her to go back up to her flat. 'They wouldn't let me leave. I was scared,' Eyakem said. 'I said, "Please, please, I just need to get my medication." They said they had been ordered not to let anyone out. They told me my medicine would be brought to me by the department, but nobody ever came.'

For days, Eyakem was too anxious to eat. She coped by holding a daily traditional African coffee ceremony in her flat with her teenage daughter. Together, they roasted raw coffee beans, stirring them over a brown clay pot. This ritual became my medicine. It was how I coped,' she said.

Inside a busy café in Fairfield in Melbourne's north, Melbourne general practitioner Ines Rio, who helped lead the public health response at the public housing towers, strained her voice over the sound of hissing coffee machines and dance music blaring from the sound system. 'I'm sorry,' she said, her eyes filling with tears, as she reflected on how the coronavirus outbreaks at the towers were handled. 'I didn't realise it was still so raw. There was just no game plan, and nobody was really held accountable.'

The day after the lockdown was announced, Rio was called early in the morning by emergency field doctors at the Flemington towers who had been sent by the government, asking her to come down to help. 'The people on the ground leading the response were just walking around looking shell-shocked and distressed,' Rio said. 'It was just chaos and utter confusion.'

Residents were calling triple zero for help. There were asthmatics with no Ventolin, diabetics without clean needles, and mothers with no nappies for their babies. But most vivid in Rio's mind years later were the agitated and anxious men, with their wide eyes and pale skin, who came down to the bottom of the towers as the early effects of methadone withdrawal kicked in. Rio said while the elderly, the women, and children stayed huddled in their flats, the desperation of these men for their next dose meant they could not be confined by police to their home. 'There were guys walking around, saying, "Please I need to get my methadone. I've got to get a pick-up",' Rio said.

Aware that some of these residents would soon be in the grips of severe withdrawal, the experienced general doctor quickly called every pharmacist in the local area, asking them who was on their methadone prescription lists. She got them to trawl their databases to find out who needed time-sensitive medication delivered. Rio also ordered dozens of pulse oximeters for the rising number of people being infected with the virus. Within about an hour, she and a few other healthcare workers at the towers had checked off the names of all the residents needing methadone. She watched the pharmacists arriving at the flats, clutching white paper bags filled with methadone prescriptions and medications.

By 23 July, nearly 350 residents in the towers had been infected with coronavirus. Like floodwaters, the virus found every crack, moving through the poorly ventilated towers into tiny flats where families of more than nine people slept. While nine towers were locked down, the majority of infections were detected in the Alfred Street flats in North Melbourne. Two of the locked-down towers did not record a single case.

Eyakem remembers the lockdown being lifted at the Flemington estate. At the stroke of midnight, elated cheers filled the towers. Hundreds of residents fled downstairs to the bottom of the flats where there is a sprawling gum tree known as the Mariam Dearit, where women meet each day; it is a reference to an ancient baobab tree in the mountainous Eritrean city of Keren, where a statue of the Madonna is located. They chanted 'We're free' under the clear, dark sky. They sang. They danced. They embraced and held each other's tear-stained faces. Eyaken said the reunion with her neighbours felt almost spiritual. 'It was so special, like this weight had been lifted from us. We were together again. We were free.'

Years later, the wounds of the lockdown lingered. Eyakem is unsure she will ever completely recover, but is doing her best to move forward. 'Life goes on. We are strong. But we will never forget.'

After delivering her report, Glass repeatedly called on the government to apologise to the 3,000 residents for the speed of the lockdown. The government has always refused to do so. Premier Daniel Andrews named the tower lockdown as 'the most challenging issue' he dealt with throughout the entire pandemic, but he said in 2021, 'What I will not do is apologise for doing everything possible to save lives— that's what we did.' Glass stressed that her findings were not a criticism of Victorian health officials who worked tirelessly and heroically to support residents and respond to the public health emergency. 'I hope the towers stand as a warning for future government decision-making and the importance of recognising the human element in everything that governments do,' Glass said during an interview in 2022. 'These were people who deserved better.'

As the hotel quarantine leak turned into a political scandal for the Andrews government, many would ask: Who hired the security guards, blamed for spreading the virus through Melbourne? Rumours circulated that the guards had been sleeping with guests and partaking in other dubious behaviour. While this made for a salacious news story, none of the gossip was proven. It was never discovered exactly how the virus got out of the hotel, but an independent inquiry by former judge Jennifer Coate, and the subsequent media reports, found that glaring infection-control problems within Victoria's early quarantine system had put staff and the Victorian community at risk.

'In particular, there were pervasive issues identified with cleaning, PPE use, and staff training and knowledge,' Coate's final report said. The Rydges hotel had no dedicated cleaning staff, so the task of cleaning common areas where Covid-positive patients had been, including the elevators, was left to general hotel staff and security. These shortfalls were magnified by the fact that Rydges had been designated as a 'hot hotel' for travellers with Covid. Problematically, the World Health Organisation was insisting at the time the quarantine system was set up that Covid-19 was primarily transmitted between people through close contact (within one metre) and off surfaces where large droplets had fallen. Airborne transmission over longer distances was considered less of a risk.

Security guards were required to do a federal government online training course that included the information that 'wearing a face mask in public won't help to protect you from infection'. They were told there was a shortage of masks, and that 'we need to save them for use when they are needed for sick people or those looking after them'. Victorian health department memos also advised that security guards did not have to wear protective equipment in hotel lobbies, or when taking guests on rooftop exercise breaks, as long as they kept a distance of 1.5 metres.

It also emerged that senior health bureaucrats initially blocked Victorian chief health officer Brett Sutton from taking control of the state's coronavirus response, against his wishes and in contradiction to the state's own pandemic plan. The-then health department deputy secretary, Melissa Skilbeck, who was later removed from her position of handling the emergency response to the pandemic, advised that Sutton would be too busy in his lead advisory role as the public face of the pandemic response to also serve as state controller overseeing the program.

Respected infectious disease expert and former federal deputy chief medical officer John Mathews would theorise that a big part of the problem with Victoria's hotel quarantine program was that Sutton did not have the attention of the premier early in the pandemic. 'Before this emergency happened, the chief health officer position in Victoria was not at a senior enough level to really have the ear of the premier,' the epidemiologist said. 'He obviously got the ear of the premier, but only when everyone realised the magnitude of the problem.'

No one would take responsibility for hiring the security guards in Victoria's quarantine hotels, or for the program's other early failings. Coate's inquiry found that police and infection-control experts should have been used in place of casual security guards. She labelled the decision to hire security guards as an 'orphan', while counsel assisting the inquiry, Rachel Ellyard, described it as a 'creeping assumption that became a reality'. One of the only clues to the origin of this decision came in a scathing 500-page final report that found the chief commissioner of police, Graham Ashton, had expressed a preference to use private security, which set off a chain of events.

In September 2020, when Andrews said that he regarded his health minister, Jenny Mikakos, as 'accountable', she had little choice but to resign. 'I have never shirked my responsibility for my department, but it is not my responsibility alone,' Mikakos said in a statement following her resignation and an excruciating day in the inquiry witness box. 'I'm deeply sorry for the situation that Victorians find themselves in. In good conscience, I do not believe that my actions led to them.' A heartbroken Mikakos would later accuse Andrews of a 'masterclass in political deflection'.

Other heads rolled, too. Health department secretary Kym Peake resigned from her role, and the state's top public servant, Chris Eccles, the secretary of the Department of Premier and Cabinet, also resigned in the wake of the scandal. The inquiry sparked an overhaul of the hotel quarantine system in Victoria but, bizarrely, did not stop most other jurisdictions from continuing to use security guards—who would be infected, alongside cleaners, again and again. By the end of the second wave in Victoria, more than 98 per cent of about 10,000 Covid cases tested had their roots in the virus's May 2020 escape from Rydges.

CHAPTER NINE

A long, dark winter

James Carlin was driving along an unusually quiet stretch of the Hume Highway, north of Melbourne, when he spotted flashing lights in the distance. He could make out orange bollards and what looked like a police breathalyser station set up alongside a service station. A police officer wearing a fluoro-yellow vest waved at him to stop. As he wound down his window, she politely requested his driver's licence and asked him his reason for travel. The owner of the Tooborac Hotel and Brewery had just dropped off a car boot load of food and leftover stock at his warehouse venue in Melbourne, fearing it would soon go to waste.

Carlin had lived all over the Middle East for seven years and had become accustomed to checkpoints there. 'But to have checkpoints in Australia? That was just unbelievably strange,' he said. 'I kept thinking *How could this be happening in our day and age in a civilised society?* Suddenly we can't travel from the city to the country.'

Several days before, on 7 July 2020, the entire city of Melbourne had been sent back into lockdown, as it became apparent the targeted shutdown of residential towers and suburbs had failed to contain a fast-moving outbreak. Nearly five million people were now unable to leave their homes for any purpose other than work or study, shopping for food and other essentials, exercise, or medical care or caregiving. Melburnians could not visit their friends or family. Restaurants and cafés opened only for takeaway.

The 'stage-three' restrictions were also extended to the Mitchell Shire, which encompassed Carlin's small country town of Tooborac, almost an hour's drive from the northern edge of suburban Melbourne. Police roadblocks were set up on arterial roads around the city to stop anyone leaving illegally, in a measure that would become known as the 'ring of steel'.

'We were just incredulous,' recalled Carlin. From the lounge-room of his rural property, with his wife and two teenage children, he had watched Victorian premier Daniel Andrews' press conference announcing the new lockdown. 'There was trepidation and fear, but also this tinge of anger of "Why are we being lumped in with the larger city suburbs of the Mitchell Shire?" There was grief about that, because it just didn't make sense to dump us all into one bucket.'

In the days that followed, Carlin loaded freshly baked pies into freezers at his hotel and brewery, which was closed due to the lockdown, and his pie shop next door, which remained open for takeaway. He opened his Carlton warehouse to a team of hospitality workers in Melbourne, who used the space to cook hundreds of meals for workers who had been laid off in Melbourne during the lockdown.

There had been 191 new cases of the disease detected in Victoria: at that point, a record high. The vast majority of infections had not yet been linked to known clusters, which was a sign that the outbreak had slipped out of the grasp of the state's public health team. Andrews, however, looked beyond his own government for blame, pointing the finger at community complacency. 'I think each of us knows someone who has not been following the rules as well as they should have been,' he said.

Melbourne's second lockdown was heralded as a 'social and economic disaster' for the city and the state. 'Sicktoria locked down for round two,' blared a headline in *The Courier-Mail* the next day. Alongside the enormous practical implications of the restrictions, there was also a sense of shame and fear that Victoria had become an outlier, suddenly isolated both psychologically and physically from the rest of the country. The other states kept their borders closed to Victoria, and moved on, largely free of the virus.

It felt like whiplash. There had been a fleeting window of freedom when Victorians could see their families again or go for a beer at the pub, only for this return to normality to be snatched away. There was collective grief when it became apparent that the new surge of cases would become another wave, and was not a speed bump on the path back to life as before.

Andrews said there was no other viable option but to bring in the sweeping lockdown. 'If we were to fail to take those steps, it won't be a couple of hundred cases a day — it will be many more than that, and it will quickly spiral well and truly out of control,' he said.

Victoria's chief health officer, Brett Sutton, told us in an interview in 2023 that Victoria's second wave of cases had snuck up on authorities, as it was hidden in the tail end of the first. 'We couldn't see there were new chains of transmission that were taking off in the way that they were,' Sutton said. 'I wish I'd acted sooner, because it would have made the scale of the challenge so much less. There were so many hard lessons like that which came after the fact about what it means not to act for a day or for a week … it means several weeks of pain and hardship and suffering, and more deaths and more disability.'

Yet epidemiologist Professor James McCaw said that his team at the University of Melbourne had been giving Victorian authorities advice to take stronger action to slow the outbreak from late June 2020, at least a week before the city-wide lockdown was announced. 'It took a lot for the premier of Victoria to act … a lot,' he said. 'The premier only acted when he acted, but the advice had been flowing for some time before that. There was a request for more certainty than could ever be provided by science, and that delayed the response. Scientists weren't able to provide the level of unambiguous "You must act" kind of advice that the premier was seeking.'

McCaw said that if Victorian authorities had gone into a citywide lockdown in late June rather than early July, the lockdown would likely have been shorter overall. However, in fairness to the officials, the mathematician also said it was only later in the pandemic that the evidence really firmed up around the benefit of acting early—that a few days' delay could translate into weeks longer in lockdown.

The first wave of coronavirus peaked in Australia at just under 460 cases a day, and more than 100 lives were lost nationally, 19 of those in Victoria. While cases in Melbourne's first wave originated from wealthy travellers returning home, including from the affluent US alpine resort of Aspen, the second wave of the virus in Victoria shifted to poorly paid, sessional security guards inside the state's hotel quarantine system before it took root in Melbourne's working-class west and north-west. It found fertile ground in those densely populated suburbs, where it crept into close-quarter workstations such as abattoirs and aged-care homes.

As the Covid count kept rising—165 cases a day, 238 cases, 459 cases—the premier's press conferences became a daily marker. For 120 consecutive days, hundreds of thousands of people tuned in via televisions, social media accounts, and news websites. Press conferences that were held early, when Andrews was dressed in his trademark North Face black jacket, signalled good news. An update late in the day, when Andrews arrived in a dark suit, foreshadowed another grim update. The press conferences often stretched out for hours as Andrews sparred with journalists until their questions were exhausted.

Professor Julian Rait, who was the Victorian president of the Australian Medical Association, said that Andrews' 'command and control' leadership, while not always popular, was what the state needed during the crisis of 2020. 'He stuck to his guns and channelled his leadership skills to make sure that everyone followed the advice that had been given to him,' Rait recalled. But he said the downside of this was that Andrews became so skilled at media management and deflection that he never really changed gears in his leadership style throughout the pandemic. 'I think as time went on, he could have been gentler in his approach,' Rait said. 'There was no real nuance in his leadership style, even during the pandemic recovery.'

During this period, Brett Sutton was spending hours each day talking through each health direction and every potential outcome in granular detail with dozens of his colleagues — from policy teams to medical advisers, public health experts, and infectious disease physicians.

'It was clear that there was a great deal of support for those decisions at that time,' Sutton said. 'It was a precautionary approach. But the general feeling was about how you needed to act when the early signs looked catastrophic, and the potential was inconceivable in many respects.'

Still, Sutton said he felt very alone as he put his signature to orders ushering in restrictions on citizens' freedom of movement, which were unprecedented in the state's living memory.

There was a heartache for Sutton being with his family physically, but not psychologically, as he tucked his young children into bed at night. 'In many respects, I didn't have a moment to contemplate how I could manage myself,' Sutton reflected. 'I wasn't thinking of it. I was thinking of all of the things that were playing out, that needed to be decided, the hundreds of emails, text messages, conversations, and meetings that were happening every day, essentially through all of 2020.'

When Sutton took his first day off in months on the anniversary of his father's death, it would happen to coincide with the day that Victoria reported its highest number of deaths in the second wave. His father, Terry, had died from a stroke when Sutton was nine years old. His death affected him deeply as a boy, to the point that Sutton was later diagnosed as being in 'profound shock' by the family's GP. Terry's death became a catalyst for him studying medicine. 'I was in my own head for a lot of that day [the anniversary], and it was particularly tough, as I recall,' Sutton said.

There were countless other difficult days, too, in the emotionally charged months of the pandemic, when chief health officers suddenly became stuck in the crossfire of politics. Sutton struggled to contain his anger after a television crew arrived at his doorstep during the lockdown of 2020, his daughter answering the door in her pyjamas. A trained emergency-medicine physician who had spent years working in refugee camps in Afghanistan, Africa, and East Timor before being drawn to public health in Victoria, he was unwittingly propelled to cult status during the pandemic. There was the public perception of him as a hero, or as the 'silver fox lining of the pandemic', and, to some, as a villain. Those of his colleagues who worked closest to him describe him as calm, thoughtful, and principled.

He described the element of celebrity that came with the job as particularly bizarre. Sutton's face was immortalised on mugs, cushions, and doona covers. Thousands of people joined a Facebook group called 'Brett Sutton is HOT', in which he was referred to as anything from the 'Dishevelled Daddy of Diseases' to our 'Chief Swoony Officer'. TikTok was swamped with videos of Australians pledging support to the state's 'CHOttie'.

'It was just really weird,' he said with a laugh. 'But I wasn't much attached to either the adulation or the vitriol. I think it is always going to happen in a crisis, to an extent, where you're a focal point of people's attention, and where the decisions do sit with you.'

Sutton said his wife, Kate, is an 'extraordinary person' who reflected back to him, lovingly yet bluntly, everything he was neglecting to do in taking care of himself. 'She was able to steward me through looking after myself in a way that maybe I couldn't do particularly well myself in 2020.' She urged him to sleep, to eat well, and to exercise. He began to run every day—something he had not done in years. He tried to take 40 minutes away from his phone each night when he could. A student of Buddhism for decades, Sutton quietened his mind by meditating. 'Intellectually, I tried to remind myself of the fact you can only do what you can do,' he said. 'If your heart and mind are in the right place to do the very best you can and with the most generous of intent, then it's hard to do much more.'

One in every 25 people who tested positive for Covid-19 in Victoria's second wave died of the virus—an excessively high mortality rate, driven by the outbreaks in aged care and by an unvaccinated population. Funeral director Andrew Pinder said that he and his colleagues were absorbing people's pain and anger as restrictions disrupted the way people grieved. 'It was the most stressful time in [living] history for funeral workers,' he reflected.

For months, each day before work, Pinder put on a tightly fitted N95 mask, foot covers, a face shield, plastic gloves, and a white hazmat suit over his collared shirt and slacks. The first of many calls to bury those infected with Covid-19 came from the tearful daughter of a man who had died alone in a Melbourne hospital in 2020. Pinder was the third funeral director the young woman had called, after the previous two had refused to dress and wash her father before his body was placed in a coffin.

'She couldn't bear the thought that her father wouldn't be dressed in his own clothing and wouldn't have that final dignity afforded to him of being clean-shaven and washed,' Pinder said. 'We ended up washing him and dressed him in his own clothing for a FaceTime viewing ceremony. Most of the man's family were infected with the virus, so a 40-minute service was held online. Even though nobody was present physically, his family phoned in from all over the world. They read letters, they cried, they told stories, and they laughed. It was really moving.'

The bodies of people who had died of Covid-19 had transparent plastic covers placed over them during services with open caskets—their skin unable to be touched by mourners. Some funeral directors stopped allowing viewings altogether because they were so fearful of catching the disease if they washed or dressed people who had died positive to Covid. Pinder, who was president of the

Australian Funeral Directors Association in 2020, said the toughest part of the job was turning distraught family members away from funerals. Limits of ten people meant that often it was the grandchildren who missed out. Any breach in protocol could have triggered a widespread ban on all funerals.

'Saying no at the chapel door to them coming inside to see their grandmother, or grieve their grandfather, goes completely against what we are in our role for,' he said. 'It was incredibly upsetting.' In late August, the premier had to intervene personally to allow a baby to be at his father's funeral because otherwise the little boy would have exceeded the ten-person cap on mourners. For some funeral directors, the toll of Melbourne's lockdowns and restrictions on funerals was too much. They took a break from the industry and never returned. 'I used to say, when someone dies, it's as hard as it gets,' Pinder said. 'But then you overlay Covid restrictions and the trauma experienced by grieving families, and it was even harder.'

Leaked documents obtained by *The Age* have suggested that there were just 14 contact tracers for the entire state of Victoria at the beginning of Australia's first wave of Covid-19 in March 2020. The state's public health unit was said to be the worst-resourced in the country. Australia's chief scientist, Professor Alan Finkel, who conducted a review of the nation's contact tracing capabilities, found that Victoria's system was only designed to manage low case numbers of infectious diseases, such as measles. Finkel noted that, for much of 2020, the state had a paper-based system and relied on contact tracers to manually enter information into an IT system. This led to duplication, cases being lost, and disastrous delays.

How Victoria's health system came to be so depleted is complicated, but many experts have blamed the devolution of the broader health system overseen by former premier Jeff Kennett and a legacy of health cuts over decades. Even in more recent times, state governments had failed to invest adequately in public health.

As the government scrambled to shore up the state's contact tracing capabilities, they brought in Professor Paul Johnson, an infectious disease doctor best known for his ground-breaking work in hunting down the mysterious Buruli ulcer, a flesh-eating infection. At the start of his first shift, on 23 July, the doctor was handed a laptop and a log-in, and joined a high-level crisis meeting led by the government's newly appointed health secretary, Professor Euan Wallace.

Days earlier, Johnson had listened to Australian scientist Dale Fisher on the radio recalling his trip to Wuhan in China for the observation mission with the World Health Organisation. The information he learnt from this would prove crucial. The Wuhan strain, which was spreading during 2020, had a serial interval of five days, which meant that every five days, on average, case numbers would triple. But Chinese authorities had found that if you got to the next exposed family before five days, and isolated and tested them, you could start to quickly squash the outbreak by getting ahead of the virus. 'My first question to the department when I got there was how long is it taking to get people who are being exposed, and the answer was, "We're so overwhelmed. Maybe seven days?"' Johnson said. 'It was clear that this time needed to be cut hugely. If you wanted to stop it, you had to go faster than it could.'

When Johnson arrived on the 13th floor of the health department's CBD headquarters, there were people in military uniforms walking around trying to help the public health team. Inside a meeting room, a long table with chairs ran down both sides, and a television screen sat at one end. Stuck all over the walls were computer-generated images of outbreaks, with coloured circles representing people, and lines connecting them to clusters.

'It felt like being in a war operations room, and there was such a sense of what was at stake at that time,' Johnson said.

Some contact tracers were in tears. 'These were exhausted people who were working like crazy. They had been trying and trying to catch up, but we had this very centralised, very under-resourced system,' Johnson said. 'Their hearts were broken.'

For Johnson, 2020 was like surfing an enormous, never-ending wave. 'It was exhilarating,' he said. The infectious disease physician worked 77 days straight. Victoria's Covid-19 response commander, Jeroen Weimar, said to him at one point, 'Look, I'm not your mother, Paul, but I think you should take a day off.' But Johnson felt a responsibility to be there for his team. 'It was deep, dark winter, and Victoria was in huge trouble,' he said. 'We were completely overrun. The other states weren't, so there was a terrible sense of loss and embarrassment as well.'

Johnson was asked by Euan Wallace to help establish localised centres, mirroring a successful New South Wales-style system made up of more than 20 public health units scattered across metropolitan and regional areas, which were deeply embedded in communities and had been built up over three decades during the AIDS crisis of the 1990s.

Within three weeks, Johnson had copied and pasted a contact tracing system already being used by Barwon Health in Geelong, and helped roll out five more Covid response units based at rural health services, from the Grampians all the way to Goulburn Valley Health. The idea was to use teams of healthcare workers based in the local area, with expert local knowledge, to hunt down the outbreaks.

He then adopted a 'mission command' approach to contact tracing based on military advice. Under this model, Victorian contact tracers were given autonomy to manage outbreaks according to a clearly articulated plan: 'Go fast, stop Covid, report back to base.'

'You had to throw old systems and rules out the window,' Johnson said. Under this system, he said, the first priority was to immediately isolate people with Covid and whoever might have come in contact with them. The next step was to get the close contacts tested and to trace the movements of the person while they were infectious.

The success of this new system would be best demonstrated a few months later in October 2020, when a Melbourne truck driver who had caught the virus from a relative working at a butcher did a cross-country road trip. The truck driver had dined illegally at

Oddfellows Café in one of Victoria's oldest inland towns, Kilmore, infecting two staff. He then made a trip to a Benalla tyre shop, White Line Tyres, and stopped in Shepparton, a city near the Goulburn River in northern Victoria. The problem behind this outbreak was that the truck driver had not told contact tracers where he had been for almost two weeks. This sent authorities into a spin, and about 20,000 people in Shepparton into isolation. Using the mission-command approach, Johnson said, a team of local nurses at the Goulburn Valley Health unit tracked down all three people infected in the outbreak within Shepparton in a single day. Their contacts were traced and quarantined, and while widespread precautionary testing followed, there were no new cases linked to that cluster.

When authorities noticed that Covid cases were falling much faster in regional areas that were using the new contact tracing approach, the government decided to roll out an identical system in three suburban public health units in Melbourne—the North Eastern, South Eastern, and Western—giving teams autonomy to manage outbreaks in their geographic areas. The first staff began working at these units in mid-December 2020. These changes completed a major overhaul of Victoria's contact tracing systems. By 2021, Victoria had built a team of more than 2,500 contact tracers and nine public health units, and had digitised its virus-tracking systems.

It was the middle of winter when Professor Allen Cheng received an unexpected phone call from health department deputy secretary Terry Symonds asking him to take on the role of deputy chief health officer at the Victorian health department. The infectious disease physician politely declined. More phone calls ensued, in which he was asked to reconsider. Then his phone lit up again. It was Australia's chief medical officer, Brendan Murphy. Cheng estimates he rejected the role about a dozen times, but after some quiet counsel at home with his wife, he had a change of heart. 'Ultimately, I felt I did have something to contribute and that I could help somehow, so I said to my wife, "Okay, we're going to do this, and it's going to be really difficult.'"

On Cheng's first day at work, on 23 July 2020, more than 400 Covid cases were reported in Victoria, partly fuelled by an outbreak at the Al-Taqwa College in Truganina in Melbourne's western suburbs, linked to more than 200 infections. At that time, it was the second-largest outbreak Australia had experienced, behind the Ruby Princess.

Cheng was convinced that in order for Victoria to have a fighting chance of coming out of lockdown, the government needed to bring in an even tougher lockdown. He said the question was 'How hard can we lock down to make it as short as possible?' to crush the outbreak and bring it down to zero cases.

With little understanding of how governments work, an enthusiastic Cheng raised his idea with premier Daniel Andrews during their first meeting. Andrew's response was blunt: 'You know, that's a billion-dollar-a-week decision. Are you really sure about that?' Cheng responded that he would 'go away and think about it a bit more'.

'I realised you don't want to just surprise the premier with something like that,' Cheng said. 'There is a whole system where you're meant to get your department to speak to his department.' Cheng described Andrews as intimidating, intense, and extraordinarily focused. 'You could tell he lived and breathed his job.'

But the premier had listened. On 2 August, Andrews announced a major escalation of restrictions that saw Melburnians largely banned from going more than five kilometres from their home, or to exercise for more than an hour a day. A state of disaster was declared, a measure intended typically for natural disasters such as bushfires. It gave the Victorian police and emergency services minister, Lisa Neville, the power to override legislation if it was in the interests of public safety. Regional Victorians also faced new movement restrictions and business closures. Until late September, each sunset in Melbourne became a warning to its residents to get home before a restrictive curfew—unprecedented in the city, even in wartime.

'We can no longer have people simply out and about for no good reason whatsoever,' Andrews said as he announced the beginning of the new restrictions. 'It is not an easy decision to make, but it is necessary, and that's why I've made it, and that's why police will be out in force, and you will be stopped and you will be asked and need to demonstrate that you are lawfully out and you are not breaching that curfew.'

Days later, cases finally started falling. The next question was, what would come next?

University of Melbourne epidemiologist Professor Tony Blakely said the orthodox view, before the Covid pandemic, had been that it was too hard to eliminate a contagion during a pandemic. But Blakely had become convinced it was the only way to go in Australia, after he and his university colleague Associate Professor Jason Thompson helped produce modelling suggesting it was possible for Victoria's outbreak to end with zero cases.

'Allen Cheng and Brett Sutton got completely on board with it,' Blakely recalled. 'They could see this was the way to go.'

Still, when Andrews announced the state's reopening plan 6 September, Father's Day, revealing that the lockdown would end only when average daily cases over the fortnight fell below five, Blakely was surprised. Sixty-three cases of Covid had been reported that day.

'I didn't think they'd be that aggressive,' Blakely observed later.

Many top epidemiologists, including Professor Jodie McVernon and Professor Mary-Louise McLaws, worried it was too stringent a goal that might never be reached. Business groups slammed the plan, and Victorian Chamber of Commerce and Industry chief executive Paul Guerra argued, 'We can't continue to let business and jobs be decimated on the way to controlling the spread of the virus.'

Prime minister Scott Morrison, along with treasurer Josh Frydenberg and health minister Greg Hunt, who represented Victorian electorates, issued a statement saying that extending lockdown arrangements would be 'hard and crushing news for the people of Victoria … The proposed roadmap will come at a further economic cost.' And just in case anyone was in doubt as to where to place the blame, the trio declared it was 'a further reminder of the impact and costs that result from not being able to contain the outbreaks of Covid-19'.

It was not the last time that the federal MPs would publicly criticise the Victorian government's record of Covid-19 management. The next month, just as the state was about to hit zero daily cases, Andrews announced that he would delay a planned announcement on the next stages of reopening by a day or two as authorities investigated a troubling outbreak in the city's north. Morrison, Hunt, and Frydenberg were swift to join the critics of the pause. 'Victoria's public health systems are either up to the task of dealing with future outbreaks or they are not,' said the trio in a joint statement.

Long-serving Labor MP Martin Foley became Victoria's health minister in September 2020 following the resignation of Jenny Mikakos. He said the outbreak, involving one of the city's African communities, needed to be sensitively managed. He was rankled by the interventions of the federal MPs, which he claimed went further than their public statements and sought to undermine the state government. He told us he had heard directly from Victorian industry leaders and others who had been personally phoned by Coalition MPs, 'saying the Victorian government's had it, they have lost control, and they're going to shut it down forever'.

Foley said he had thought a lot about whether Morrison would have preferred Victoria to have failed in containing the second wave because of the damage it would have done to the state's Labor government. 'I can't in my mind's eye imagine a position where the federal government would want that to be the case, yet every piece of evidence tells me that they are having a schizophrenic process of, on the one hand, inadequately supporting [Victoria] where they could, and, on the other hand, adopting that let's-tear-down-Victoria stance,' he said. 'It was bizarre, bad politics, let alone very bad public policy.'

The Australian Capital Territory's chief minister, Andrew Barr, said the closest that national cabinet came to blowing up was in May 2020, after one of Morrison's MPs, education minister Dan Tehan, appeared on the ABC's political panel-show *Insiders* and accused Andrews of a 'failure of leadership' for keeping schools closed. 'I think the accusation was made that Morrison was using his ministers as bomb-throwers, essentially,' said Barr. 'In terms of the dynamics of the room, it was pretty palpable at that point, [that] unless the attack dogs were reined in, Morrison and Andrews weren't able to work together.' Tehan, a Victorian MP, later said that he had overstepped the mark in questioning Andrews' leadership.

Come late September 2020, Allen Cheng said that health officials were also feeling the pressure from a frustrated public, agitating for more freedoms. But the epidemiologist's lingering fear was that coronavirus cases could soar again if Victoria reopened too fast, and that it would be almost impossible to ask weary residents to repeat a prolonged lockdown. 'We only really had one shot at reopening,' Cheng said. 'If we opened up at 50 [cases] and then went up to 200 again, we would be in all sorts of trouble.'

It was around this time, as Cheng walked nervously into Treasury Place for another gruelling coronavirus press conference, that Andrews turned and told him that 1.5 million people were tuned in to watch the daily briefing. The premier was unfazed. Cheng almost tripped over the stairs into the lecture theatre. 'I thought, *Oh my God, how many people are going to be watching what I say?*'

Vignettes stand out for Cheng from that time: quiet moments reading Harry Potter with his children; his children's laughter as they ran around the house in the background during Zoom calls with the premier; sitting down to dinner with his family moments before the phone rang again with news of another outbreak and more deaths; and mapping out his daily 59-minute jog when the five-kilometre radius was enforced, careful not to break the rules, which at the time allowed for only an hour of exercise.

On 26 October 2020, Victoria reported zero cases for the first time in close to 20 weeks. It would become the first of many 'doughnut days'. (The term was inspired by the rounded shape of the fried treat, like a zero.) The next day, pubs and restaurants across

Melbourne flung open their doors as the clock ticked past midnight and lockdown rules were officially eased. Thirsty Melburnians clamoured for a long-awaited pint.

Cheng estimates that roughly 10,000 and 20,000 people could have died in Victoria in 2020 if the outbreak had been left to spread. At the end of July, just before Melbourne's second wave reached its peak, France, the UK, and Australia were reporting a very similar number of daily Covid-19 cases. By August, Melbourne's second wave was on the downward trajectory, but cases in the UK and France were mounting. England would peak at around 70,000 daily cases and more than 1,000 daily deaths the following January, as the country entered its third national lockdown. France had hundreds of daily deaths by late 2020. Victorians, meanwhile, were able to enjoy an almost normal summer (excluding a 'circuit-breaker' five-day lockdown in February).

The difference? 'We made the decision to lock down early, and they didn't,' Cheng said.

CHAPTER TEN

How could this happen in Australia?

Memories of old people lying in beds, delirious and burning up with fever, remain raw in Mark Murray's mind. When coronavirus found its way into aged-care homes during Victoria's dark winter of 2020, Murray's phone would light up at night. Another aged-care facility was in crisis and dangerously understaffed. He would dress quickly in his personal protective gear: a tightly fitted face mask that dug painfully into his skin, a scrub cap, a face shield, and a gown. Then he was off, driving to whichever aged-care facility in the west needed him.

The experienced nurse at Western Health attended about a third of all outbreaks at residential aged-care facilities in Australia in the first two years of the pandemic. 'That's how big the outbreak was in the west of Melbourne,' Murray said during a phone interview from his home in December 2022. He had just caught coronavirus for the first time, and was isolating. 'We were caring for one-third of residents in aged care who had coronavirus, and dealing with a third of the deaths. I have been doing this for 15 years. It was death at a scale that I had never, ever seen before.'

If the true measure of a society is how it treats its least powerful members, then Australia tragically failed many of its elderly citizens in residential aged care in the first few years of the coronavirus pandemic. For every three aged-care residents infected with the virus in Victoria in 2020, roughly one of them died. There were no vaccines or antiviral treatments available, and it quickly became clear that no other survival factor mattered as dramatically as age. Those who were older were more likely to have underlying conditions, such as diabetes or heart and lung disease, that made their bodies more vulnerable to Covid. Our immunity also wanes as we get old, and doctors suspect the process of ageing can trigger a phenomenon called a cytokine storm, where the immune system overreacts when threatened by a virus. This can lead to organ failure.

Safety measures, such as strict visitor restrictions, imposed in Australia's aged-care facilities slowed the devastation at first. During the first wave of the Covid-19 pandemic in 2020, three residents caught the virus in Victorian public sector aged-care homes, and all survived. But between March and December that same year, there were more than 2,000 coronavirus cases in aged-care homes, and 655 residents died across 50 homes. At St Basil's, 45 of the home's 117 residents—with an average age of 85—died of Covid-19 within a month. Thirty-four residents at Epping Gardens aged-care facility died after contracting Covid-19, and at Kalyna Care in Delahey, 23 of its 102 residents died after being infected.

Independent reviews of the outbreaks at Epping Gardens and St Basil's would find that both facilities had poor emergency planning, inadequate staff training, and insufficient infection-prevention and control procedures. Once Covid escaped Victoria's hastily assembled hotel quarantine, it quickly began to circulate in the community, infecting thousands of essential and casual workers, including poorly paid personal-care assistants and aged-care workers who were working shifts in multiple homes to make ends meet.

Professor Joseph Ibrahim sensed in late February that a crisis in aged care was on the horizon. Ibrahim, who is one of Australia's top aged-care experts, was desperately trying to get an opinion piece published in a major news outlet, warning that urgent action needed to be taken to protect the elderly. No media outlet was interested in publishing it, he said. He tried writing to senior health officials, including the federal aged-care minister, Richard Colbeck, to no avail. In the end, he started his own podcast to try to get the word out.

'I felt angry and frustrated that nobody was really listening or asking the questions of politicians, and there seemed to be no interest in helping or preparing aged care for what inevitably came,' said Ibrahim, a professor at the Australian Centre for Evidence Based Aged Care at La Trobe University in Melbourne. 'Homer Simpson could have seen the catastrophe in aged care coming with Covid-19, because it was right there in your face.'

What troubles the families of aged-care residents who died in Victoria's second wave most is that, only months earlier, a corona-virus outbreak at Newmarch House in western Sydney was linked to the deaths of 19 elderly residents. The failures at Newmarch House should have been a warning for the rest of the country to act. The facility's hospital-in-the-home approach was found to have been 'compromised by inadequate staffing', and the families of the people who died said they were discouraged from taking their loved ones out of the facility. In a searing final report on the outbreak in August 2020, infectious disease physician Professor Lyn Gilbert and health and aged-care consultant Alan Lilly, who examined the fail-ings, described the leadership of Anglicare, Newmarch's operator, as being 'generally invisible to external parties interacting with them'. They found it ultimately justified the intervention of the Aged Care Quality and Safety Commission.

At 76, Ann Fahey was one of the youngest residents at the Newmarch House aged-care home when she died. She collapsed on the floor of her room 19 days after the first case was detected, and died in hospital soon after on 2 May. Ann was a bubbly, social, and intelligent woman who had moved into Newmarch House, not because of healthcare needs or any deterioration of her mind, but because she no longer wanted to live on her own. Her death devas-tated her granddaughter Nicole Fahey and her only son, Mark. Fahey said Mark now struggled with post-traumatic stress disorder and had been left riddled with guilt over his mother's death. 'To see people in Victoria go through what we did months later was just gut-wrenching and despicable. Neither the federal nor state governments had learnt the lessons,' Fahey said. 'They just let it happen all over again. We want the true story to be told so this Australian aged-care disaster is never allowed to occur again.'

There was none worse in Australia than the outbreak at St Basil's Home for the Aged in Fawkner in Melbourne's northern suburbs. It was inside this facility, owned and managed by the Greek Orthodox Church, that conditions during an outbreak in the winter of 2020 deteriorated to the point that starving residents tried to bash down the centre's front door to escape the chaos and find food. The outbreak was Australia's deadliest. On top of the 45 who died from Covid, another five residents also died, allegedly due to neglect.

Many residents were malnourished and dehydrated. They were left without their medication for days. The kitchen at St Basil's ran out of food as 80 per cent of residents, and most of the 120 staff, were infected. Frail residents were left in soiled bedding and clothing, some covered in painful pressure sores or bed wounds. One experienced nurse would tell a five-week inquest examining the handling of the outbreak that a pressure sore she treated on a resident during the outbreak was unlike anything she had seen in the two decades of her career. 'It hadn't been dressed, and it looked nasty. You were able to see into the wound and see the tendons,' she said.

The extent of the neglect and horror that unfolded inside St Basil's was perhaps best described by Kirsten Congerton, a consultant employed by the Victorian health department, who volunteered to visit St Basil's to assist with the response on 23 July 2020. In an email sent at 4.41 the following morning to a health department official, Congerton wrote:

> St Basil's was horrific. I cried several times on site and I'm pretty tough. We had one person pass away, we expect two or

three more overnight. They have written many residents off as palliative. The place is a mess. It is not stable or improving ... We had to manage the staff ... [no managers] were in a condition to psychologically do so ... PCA [personal-care assistants] in tears, RN [registered nurse] in over their heads and obviously frightened. There were no stations for nurses or carers to remove their personal protective equipment, or bins to put waste into. We had to resort to tying bags outside residents' rooms so the very young, inexperienced, terrified, and overwhelmed agency staff could doff [remove their PPE]. Clients not being fed, meds missed, hygiene unattended, in their nappies for hours and hours. Bed sores ... [another employee] and I have seen a lot in our time and experience, but this is horrific for everyone involved.

Jayne Erdevicki had been trying desperately for days to get news about her 82-year-old father, Boro, who had been living in St Basil's for two years. Each time she called, the phone would ring out. Finally, a call came just before midnight one evening in late July. 'I'm just calling to let you know your father's gone,' a woman's voice said. In the backyard of her home in Werribee on a warm spring afternoon more than two years later, Erdevicki struggled to relive the moment. 'I lost it, I started crying,' she said. 'I said: "Why didn't anybody call? Why didn't anybody call? I've been ringing and ringing."' Her face contorted with sorrow and anguish at the memory of that night, and her eyes filled with tears. 'She [the caller] said, "You need to take him out of here. We need somebody to pick up the body." It was like he was just a piece of rubbish. *Come collect the rubbish and throw it out.'*

Erdevicki was told by St Basil's management that her father had died of coronavirus, but a coroner would later find that Boro, a Yugoslavian migrant who had come to Australia to build a better life for his family, was not infected at the time of his death. The exact cause of his death remains unknown. Erdevicki suspects that neglect played a role. At night, she has nightmares of running through dark, empty corridors, opening doors, trying to find her father. She has not watched the news for more than three years. Any mention of the coronavirus pandemic, or even just the sound of Victorian premier Daniel Andrews' voice, is enough to cause her to shake with rage or break down in tears.

'When it comes to St Basil's, I am lost for words,' said Erdevicki, who was part of a group of families pursuing a class action against the operators of St Basil's at the time of this book's publication. 'How could this happen in Australia? How could people be so inhumane? These were the people who were meant to protect them.'

Melbourne funeral director Andrew Pinder had spent his life surrounded by the dead. From the age of ten he worked through his school holidays helping out at the family business, fitting the fabric lining inside coffins and nailing on the handles, before bodies were placed inside. Yet nothing prepared him for what he was confronted with at St Basil's and other aged-care homes in Melbourne's northern suburbs, where he travelled to collect the bodies of the dead in 2020. 'It was a record number of deaths in a short period of time,' Pinder said.

The only other event in modern history that came close to the scale of death he and his colleagues experienced during this time was the 2009 Black Saturday bushfires, when 173 people perished. Some days, when Pinder arrived at St Basil's in his silver transfer van fitted out with hydraulic equipment to transport a body, the media presence outside was so intense that he would leave. He wanted to afford the dead privacy and dignity, and would return late in the day when the journalists and television crews had dispersed. The process for retrieving the bodies involved gently placing a mask or a small cloth on their face before shifting them from their bed to a gurney. There was a fear that if oxygen was trapped in their lungs, it could be released when they were moved. 'It was possible for virus particles to become airborne if there was exhalation by the deceased, so we covered their faces to protect ourselves,' Pinder said.

Sometimes Pinder would be asked by families to pick up the bodies of deceased aged residents from a temporary morgue that had been set up at the Royal Melbourne Hospital's Royal Park campus in Parkville. Several refrigerated shipping containers, containing mortuary racks for bodies, and hydraulic trolleys to avoid manual handling, sat for weeks in a car park outside the hospital. The morgue was cordoned off by industrial fencing and concealed behind black fabric that was wrapped around the metal fencing to preserve the privacy of the dead. He would transport the bodies into his van and take them to his mortuary in Preston. When he came home at night and turned on the television news, footage of St Basil's would flash on the screen. 'It was all so strange,' he said. 'The word I kept using at the time was cruel. It was so cruel for families to be apart from their dying loved ones.'

The 54-year-old runs Ern Jensen Funerals, which has parlours in Preston and St Albans. He said that his staff held dozens of funerals for aged-care residents during the crisis. The grief of families was often intensified by chaotic conditions inside the homes, which meant that their loved ones' paperwork, including their death verification forms, were sometimes missing. Pinder said at times there was even confusion about where bodies were and whether they had been picked up. 'We were sent to homes, only to be told the body had already been picked up and taken to a morgue,' he said.

The father of one of his colleagues died during an outbreak at an aged-care home in Altona. Unable to be with his father, the man kept a vigil in the car park for two days, in the rain and through the night, refusing to leave until his dad died. 'Imagine not even being able to be in the same room as your loved one, so you're standing outside in a car park in the rain so that they don't die alone?' Pinder said. 'I can't imagine what that must have been like. That is something that has never left me.'

As Clay Lucas from *The Age* reported in 2021, St Basil's was full of elderly migrants who had built modern Australia in the years after World War II. Among those who died in the outbreak were bus drivers, welders, fish-and-chip shop owners, mechanics from the Ford factory in Broadmeadows, and seamstresses. None of the residents who died between 21 July and 23 August in 2020 were born in Australia, and many relied heavily on their carers in the aged-care home due to language barriers.

The outbreak at St Basil's began when an infected personal-care assistant came to work. She was unaware she had Covid-19, and wasn't showing any symptoms. The woman lived with her extended family in one of the ten local government areas that had been ordered into lockdown by the Victorian government on 30 June 2020. After finishing work on 5 July, she drove to a nearby drive-through testing clinic, and was swabbed for the virus. But on the advice of a senior registered nurse at St Basil's, she continued to go to work while waiting for her result, working two full shifts on 6 and 7 July. The following day, she was at work again when she received a text from her husband that the family had all tested positive. She left work immediately. By then, the virus had already seeded inside the home. Staff would not be told about the positive case until a week later, on 14 July.

When things deteriorated inside St Basil's, it happened quickly. But, as *The Age* detailed in its editorial, it would take just the first day of the inquest probing the disaster for Peter Rozen KC and assisting state coroner John Cain to lay out in distressing detail just how many failures of process had occurred in such a short time at St Basil's. By 24 July 2020, about 19 days after the first infected staff member had a Covid test, Rozen said 'the true extent of the neglect became apparent to those at the highest levels of the Commonwealth and Victorian governments'. It was on this day that Dr Luis Prado, chief medical officer of the Epworth Hospital, visited St Basil's, immediately ordering residents to be given the care they urgently needed in a hospital.

For many residents, it was already too late. Workers would describe chaotic scenes of overflowing bins, medicine strewn on the floor, and a dead body being wheeled down the corridor in full view of residents. Scenes captured by media outlets outside St Basil's Home for the Aged and outside Epping Gardens remain the most harrowing of the entire pandemic in Australia. Old people, frightened and wide-eyed, wrapped in blankets, many on the brink of death, were taken out on gurneys and wheelchairs by masked healthcare workers into rows of waiting ambulances. Laid out on other stretchers were the bodies of the dead, hidden under blankets and concealed in zipped-up body bags. It would take ten days for authorities to evacuate St Basil's after the first resident died with coronavirus.

Con Velissaris was 79 when he caught the virus in St Basil's. Television crews captured him lying on a stretcher being wheeled out by healthcare workers in white hazmat suits before he was put into the back of an ambulance and transferred to Glenferrie Private Hospital. Velissaris, who is the only resident of St Basil's to speak publicly to the media about his experience, was haunted by the sounds of terrified staff screaming in the halls. 'The last four or five days, nurses were screaming and running around, so many people were dying,' he told Nine News in 2021. 'People die now, they die later, everyday one of them dies.' He credited the staff at Glenferrie Private Hospital with saving his life.

As the outbreak unravelled at St Basil's, distraught families gathered outside the aged-care facility, nestled in a sprawling three hectares of grassland scattered with fruit trees on the edge of the Merri Creek. They began banging on the windows before being threatened by staff. 'One of the nurses came out and they said, if you don't stop that, we're going to call the police,' said Christine Golding, whose mother, Efraxia Tsalanidis, died at St Basil's in 2020. 'I do remember someone called the police, the Fawkner police department. He said our parents are kept prisoner there. The neglect that my mother suffered at St Basil's was inhumane, cruel, and degrading.'

It would be profoundly unfair to place blame on what unfolded at St Basil's on any single individual. Instead, what occurred was a cascade of catastrophic failures at every level, at the heart of which was the entrenched systemic ineptitude that has long plagued the aged-care sector. Joseph Ibrahim, who has worked for more than 30 years in geriatric medicine, said there was confusion over responsibility between federal and state governments, a regulator that failed to see a disaster coming, delays in care and infection control, and severe worker shortages. Everything deficient about aged care in Australia and how we care for the elderly in the final years of their lives was exposed, he said.

As the Royal Commission into Aged Care Quality and Safety stated in its interim report in 2019: 'As a nation, Australia has drifted into an ageist mindset that undervalues older people and limits their possibilities. We have found that the aged-care system ... does not deliver uniformly safe and quality care for older people. It is unkind and uncaring towards them. In too many instances, it simply neglects them.' Aged care in Australia is predominantly regulated and funded by the federal government. About 95 per cent of St Basil's $13 million in annual income came from federal government grants. The Greek Orthodox Church, which oversees St Basil's, was also paid millions of dollars annually in rent by the facility in the five years before the pandemic.

Professor Ibrahim said the pandemic revealed deep fractures between the state and federal governments' responsibilities and roles. Confusion and incoordination within the emergency response caused unnecessary deaths, he said. Ibrahim said those in aged care were failed on many fronts: by governments, politicians, the aged-care sector, and the industry regulator, the Aged Care Quality and Safety Commission. 'They all pretty much sang from the same hymn book ... that it was all under control and everyone was working together, but the reality was very different,' he said.

While the federal government was largely responsible for aged care, providing almost $15 billion per year in funding to cover the costs of personal and health care for residents, the Victorian government was responsible for outbreak management and access to acute hospital care. It was for this reason that an inquiry into St Basil's would heavily scrutinise a decision by Victoria's chief health officer,

Brett Sutton, to stand down all the home's staff. This furloughing of all the home's staff was ordered following advice from the former senior medical adviser at the Department of Health, Dr Finn Romanes, and was based on the assumption that a surge workforce would be brought in by the federal government.

What was unknown to Sutton at the time was that the very same day this advice was acted upon, there were warnings from two senior doctors on the ground that the outbreak would be disastrous for residents. A senior Northern Hospital doctor, Sandra Brown, whose team visited the home during this period, warned Victorian department of health officials in an email of 'residents starving to death and dying of dehydration from basic care needs not being met'. Brown said that either St Basil's Covid-negative staff should be brought back to the home to care for the residents, or the army needed to be brought in.

Northern Hospital geriatrician Zi Yi Low also raised her fears for St Basil's residents after assisting in an earlier Covid-19 outbreak at an Estia aged-care home in Heidelberg, where ten people died and staff had also been stood down. 'Medications were lost, meals were not provided, no modified diet or fluids and no analgesia,' Dr Low was recorded as saying in a police brief prepared for the coroner. She warned that 'if St Basil's goes down this path, a facility triple the size of Estia Heidelberg—this will be disastrous.'

The inquiry would find that the hasty transition to a replacement management team and surge workforce was not sustainable. Sutton said senior staff from his department had not alerted him to concerns held by Commonwealth staff and doctors that pulling together a replacement workforce would be nearly impossible, or that they feared residents would be left without basic care, including food and medications.

Knowing how infectious the virus was and how quickly it spread, the public health physician said he and other officials were left with 'an extraordinarily difficult set of risks to balance'. There were awful trade-offs in the provision of care and welfare against the risk of transmission, Sutton said. But he had been terrified that the spread would have been even more significant if the original staff had been allowed to stay on site. By the time Sutton had signed the order to stand down the entire workforce, there were at least 50 positive cases connected to the home. Sutton later told the inquiry he believed the refusal by the former manager of St Basil's aged-care home, Kon Kontis, and the director of nursing, Vicky Kos, to immediately accept the furlough direction from the Victorian health department may have led to more cases of the virus in the home.

The nation's chief nursing officer, Alison McMillan, was also caught up in the crisis. McMillan visited St Basil's at the request of Australia's chief medical officer, Brendan Murphy, and aged-care minister, Richard Colbeck—something that she, too, would face scrutiny over during the inquiry. McMillan initially advised against a mass evacuation of the 117 residents as regular workers were sent home and replaced by inexperienced agency staff, just over a week before the aged-care facility was shut down. Her advice came hours after the first death from coronavirus. The deaths did not stop for a month. In November 2021, McMillan would be questioned in the coroner's court about her advice and the fact that she had not checked on residents in their rooms.

'Would you think it appropriate, now knowing what you do, to at least walk around the facility and have a look and see some of the residents?' state coroner John Cain asked McMillan during the inquest. 'With the benefit of hindsight, absolutely,' she replied.

It was an experience that took a personal toll on McMillan. She told us later that she was home in Melbourne from Canberra one weekend when she received a call from Professor Paul Kelly, then Australia's deputy chief medical officer, asking her to spend a few days helping the Victorian health department, who 'were really stretched'. McMillan said her role when she visited St Basil's was to ensure that replacement staff had been arranged, and that those staff had turned up for work. When she arrived and spent the morning at the facility, she observed that the surge staff were there, being orientated and being given areas of responsibility to care for residents.

That evening, McMillan was involved in setting up the Victorian Aged Care Response Centre, bringing together state and federal officials to try to manage the outbreak and the others that they expected to occur. McMillan said she was among many who had underestimated what a Covid outbreak in a residential aged-care facility might mean. 'We had plans. We had provided material and training. We provided PPE. But perhaps [we] hadn't anticipated the magnitude of the challenge, and that there would be so many at the same time,' she said. 'We were seeing [the number] of outbreaks double every two days in those following weeks.'

In late July, Victoria's health department ordered anyone who had worked at St Basil's and had been there within a two-week period to be declared a close contact and quarantined. This move meant that the entire workforce needed to be replaced with agency staff by 22 July. Aspen Medical, a contractor whose staff were not familiar with the residents, was brought in by the federal government. The private nursing contractor was paid millions by the government to supply the temporary replacement workforce, but was unable to secure enough competent carers. The workers it did secure got infected, too.

Some Aspen contractors left their first shift so traumatised by what they saw that they simply refused to return again, saying the conditions were appalling, *The Age* reported. Even the company's deputy head of nursing chose not to return after his first shift, fearing he would lose his nursing registration. The Aspen staff who stayed on, including nurse Jacinta MacCormack, made valiant efforts to care for the residents. 'I was here in this war zone, and I just did what I thought was right at the time,' MacCormack, who had been a nurse for more than 40 years, told investigators in 2021. 'There were patients that were obviously malnourished as well as dehydrated. There was a couple that actually looked quite emaciated. Their hips were sticking out.'

The coroner's inquest never laid blame at the feet of the workers who were brought in and courageously risked their lives to take care of the residents. Instead, it found that there were far too few of these workers at St Basil's for them to have ever provided care at the level the residents deserved and the law required. 'They were operating within a wholly inadequate governance and management structure trying to look after over 100 frail, elderly people, many of whom were suffering from a deadly and highly infectious disease. If anything, the evidence will reveal that a number of the replacement staff went above and beyond.'

Mark Murray saw the best in humanity reflected in the efforts of his colleagues from Western Health, who did everything they could to save lives during the dozens of outbreaks at aged-care facilities they attended in the city's western suburbs. Starting his own career as a poorly paid personal-care assistant earning about $20 an hour, Murray said his heart had broken for the aged-care staff, who he felt had no option but to go along with the organisational decisions and the policy-making of the aged-care facilities that they worked for at that time.

'Much has been learnt since then. But there was no policy or system in place that was able to deal with what we dealt with,' he said. It was a crisis, he believes, complicated by the fact that there were no legislated minimum ratios of nursing staff to residents in private and not-for-profit aged care at that time. 'I don't have rose-coloured glasses on. I know that there were some terrible things happening in aged-care facilities, and things that could have well been avoided,' Murray said. 'But at the same time, there was an overwhelming struggle. A lot of the staff on the ground were getting blamed for things when it's exactly the same as blaming a bank teller for rising interest rates on mortgages. You're blaming people with no authority or power.'

When Murray reflects on this period, it is the isolation and what he describes as the 'unintentional neglect' of residents during coronavirus outbreaks in aged care—such as those going without water, or being severely unwell and not having somebody with them holding their hand—that still hurts him most. It went against everything he believed in as a nurse. Staff did their best to gently comfort the residents. Some even took to filling latex gloves with warm water, and putting them under the hands of the elderly—the idea being that the warmth of the glove could replicate the hand of a loved one, and make them feel less alone. He recalled one feverish woman who was just lying quietly and very still in her bed in an aged-care home in Melbourne's western suburbs before she died. 'It was just terrible. It was almost like her deterioration was getting missed because she was so quiet,' he said.

He remembers telling another woman late one evening that her mother was dying of coronavirus. 'The reason that sticks with me so much was because that poor woman was devastated, absolutely devastated, and she was unable to come into the facility,' Murray said. 'Through her grief she was thanking me for what I could do and for being there. I just thought, *This is such a terrible thing. I should be in the same room with this person. We should be both together. She should be able to be with her mum.*'

One of the final times that Jayne Erdevicki saw her dad, she was unable to go inside the aged-care facility due to visitor restrictions. The father and daughter were left staring at each through a double-glazed glass door at St Basil's. The months of near-isolation had taken a toll on Boro, and Jayne recalls being shaken by her father's appearance. He had lost weight, and his eyes were hollow and distant. His cheekbones were protruding out of the pale skin on his face, and he looked malnourished. When Boro realised Jayne was standing outside, he curled up his fists and started banging on the door, howling to be close to his daughter. 'I broke down. I got in the car and I just sat there bawling my eyes out. I couldn't drive. I couldn't move,' Jayne said.

For many elderly people, their final months or years were spent suffering through the pandemic. Renowned aged-care activist Merle Mitchell summed it up succinctly when she told the royal commission into aged care in 2020 that she woke up every day disappointed to be alive. 'I know I'm here until I die, so every morning when I wake up I think, *Damn, I've woken up.*' The 85-year-old, who died the following year, had been stuck in her room inside a Glen Waverley nursing home in Melbourne for months, other than for her four physiotherapy sessions. 'Otherwise, from the time I wake up to the time I go to sleep, I'm sitting in my own room in my one chair,' she said. 'It is not to say I'm not being cared for, but I am sure if you asked most people here, they would all say they would rather be dead, rather than living more, if they're honest.'

Without a national inquiry probing the aged-care response during the pandemic, Professor Ibrahim remained concerned that the lessons of St Basil's and other homes were yet to be applied in Australia in a meaningful way. By the end of 2022, more than 4,000 Australians in residential aged care had died with coronavirus. When the infectious Omicron variant emerged just before Christmas 2021, an average of 17 residents were dying every day, despite many of them being vaccinated by then. The vast majority had underlying illnesses, mostly dementia, and their leading cause of death was pneumonia. For those who were immunised when they died, it remains difficult to determine just how much of a contributing factor coronavirus was in their deaths. But for the hundreds of unvaccinated Victorians who perished in the aged-care outbreaks of 2020, their final moments were filled with confusion, chaos, and loneliness.

'There were human rights abuses, these were people arguably living out the end of their lives, but they did not need to die like that … in conditions so awful,' Ibrahim said. 'Their agency over their own bodies was robbed from them and from their families. If we want the world to be a better place, then how we treat older people would really be an example of how we should be treating each other.'

CHAPTER ELEVEN

South Australia, the quiet achiever

South Australia's chief public health officer, Nicola Spurrier, knew as soon as she was woken by her phone buzzing in the early hours one Saturday morning that the news she was about to hear was unwelcome. It was the same sort of feeling she had had while on call as a paediatrician earlier in her career, when she was certain that the emergency on the other end of the line was 'going to be a child with meningitis, or something bad'. This particular night in November 2020, an 81-year-old woman had arrived at the Lyell McEwin Hospital in Adelaide's sprawling northern suburbs feeling a little weak and 'off'. Until she coughed, there was little about the woman's symptoms that indicated she had Covid-19. As a precaution, a junior doctor named Dharminy Thurairatnam had ordered a respiratory illness test, and it had delivered a shock positive result.

Steven Marshall, the South Australian premier, remembers receiving the notification on that Saturday 14 November. It was the first case of coronavirus detected in South Australia outside the confines of hotel quarantine for many months. From a small conference room at his electorate office on the main street of Norwood, an affluent inner-city suburb of Adelaide well known for its cafés and boutique stores, Marshall remembers that by the time the outbreak was detected, the virus was already on the run and on its way to some of the places where it would be most dangerous.

'We immediately contacted all of her close contacts, and a high proportion of them had [Covid]. Those close contacts worked in aged care, the prison system, and the mines. It was very fortuitous that we didn't have an explosion off that single case,' he said. It took a couple of days, but the cluster triggered the first of South Australia's two 'short but sharp' state lockdowns, making national and international headlines.

Professor Spurrier was very worried about certain 'characteristics' of the strain of coronavirus detected. 'It has a very, very short incubation period. That means when someone gets exposed, it's taken 24 hours or even less for that person to become infectious to others,' she explained in a press conference. '[Cases have] had minimal symptoms and sometimes no symptoms, but have been able to pass it on to other people.'

Critical to the management of the outbreak was the involvement of a pizza shop in the western suburb of Woodville. There was a confirmed case at the venue: one of many similar small family-owned stores like it in Australia, on a busy main road, serving Hawaiian pizza and chicken supreme. Spurrier's team were so anxious about the possibility that Covid-19 had spread to customers of the store that they asked everyone who had ordered takeaway from the Woodville Pizza Bar to go into quarantine for 14 days. And a six-day 'circuit breaker' lockdown was announced, with some of the strictest coronavirus rules seen in Australia: exercise outside the house was banned; only essential food services could operate; and even takeaway was excluded. Just about everything was closed. Among the limited exceptions were banks, bottle shops, and medical services.

When we spoke to Professor Spurrier about this period, it was via video chat, and the pandemic was in its third year. We had arranged to meet her earlier in Adelaide, but the meeting had been cancelled when a media officer from SA Health called to tell us what we had already read on several news sites: the 'top public health doctor' had a mild dose of coronavirus. 'It's a bit hard when all your health ends up in the paper.' Spurrier smiles warmly as she talks, explaining she had been inspired by New Zealand in her approach to the 'couple of little outbreaks here in our state'.

'I'd seen what had happened in Victoria and New South Wales, and I didn't want that to happen to people in my state, so that's why we had these short, sharp lockdowns,' she said. 'I'm sure people thought, *God, she's totally over the top, she won't even let us go out of the house for a walk.* But I only wanted it for a short time, because I had a really hot contact tracing team, and I knew that if given three or six days, however long it took, they [would] be able to find every single case ... get their close contacts, get their secondary close contacts ... get them all into quarantine, and then I'll be okay to [lift the lockdown].'

In the end, the planned six-day lockdown only lasted three days. In an explosive press conference on 20 November, Marshall said the decision to go into lockdown had been based on a lie. A man allegedly told contact tracers he had caught coronavirus after purchasing a pizza from the pizza bar, prompting authorities to become worried about the possibility that he may have caught the virus off a pizza box. 'The information that came back from the contact tracers was that this was a *customer* of a fast-food outlet. We thought, *Well, wow, how virulent, how transmissible, how dangerous is this strain?,*' Marshall told us later. 'As it turned out, that person was working alongside somebody else, who had it. It was a completely different equation ... instead of [having] tens and tens and tens of thousands of people we would have to contact trace, it actually was a much smaller number.'

The man, a Spanish national, had worked at the shop for several shifts alongside an infectious hotel quarantine security guard, meaning he'd had ample opportunity to pick up the virus from the guard. Marshall could barely contain his rage when he announced the news, accompanied by an immediate easing of restrictions. He accused the man of having deliberately misled contact tracers, and blamed him for the lockdown. 'To say I am fuming about the actions of this individual is an absolute understatement,' Marshall said. 'The selfish actions of this individual have put our whole state in a very difficult situation. His actions have affected businesses, individuals, family groups, and is completely and utterly unacceptable.'

Many others also directed their anger at the man and his blameless employer, Sam Norouzi, the owner of the pizza bar in Woodville at the centre of it all. Norouzi later told *The Advertiser* that he had received death threats, and that pictures of his baby and his private telephone number were posted on Facebook. Police were stationed at the store to ward off potential vigilante attacks. Hundreds of angry South Australians bombarded the Facebook page and Google listing of the fast-food outlet with negative comments and reviews. 'You willingly and willfully lied,' one person wrote. 'You caused an entire state to go into lockdown. You caused many casual staff to lose income. You should be ashamed of yourselves.'

It was one of many times in the pandemic when small actions of ordinary people were blamed for coronavirus lockdowns, and when their blunders or rule-breaking were monumentally magnified. Years later, South Australia's own 'pizzagate' was what people remembered about this outbreak of 33 detected cases. Fewer recalled that the outbreak was the result of the coronavirus managing to make its way from a British guest in a quarantine hotel in Adelaide, spreading first to a security guard and cleaner, and then outwards into the community. This was the first time, publicly at least, that problematic ventilation in hotels was implicated by authorities in an outbreak. An investigation by SA Health published in mid-January the next year found that the infected guest had opened their door while not wearing a mask while one of the security guards and the cleaner were in the corridor nearby.

Still, 'pizzagate' and another outbreak in July the following year were rare disruptive blips in a long period that South Australia enjoyed between the initial national lockdown that ended in May 2020 and the Omicron wave that began at Christmas the next year. In that time, the state spent just ten days in lockdown. It was as if the pandemic didn't exist.

Along with Marshall and Spurrier, there was a third key figure in South Australia's Covid response: police commissioner Grant Stevens. When a major emergency declaration was made in the state in March 2020, Stevens was installed as the state's coronavirus coordinator. It was a decision that effectively elevated him to the position of 'leader of the state', said Andrew Hough, *The Advertiser*'s chief pandemic correspondent. Stevens was charged with making monumental decisions around lockdowns and border closures. The emergency declaration had only been used for bushfires and severe weather events about half a dozen times in South Australia's history, and only for up to about four days at a time. Never had it needed to be extended. During the pandemic, it remained in place for 793 days, and was extended 28 times.

Stevens disputes that he became the state's unelected leader, saying that there had been more to running the state than just Covid-19. Yet the significance of the enormous power and responsibility he was granted, and the impact of the decisions he made, is not lost on him. 'This is the first time ever that I was making decisions that impacted on the entire state,' he said. 'People were having to close their businesses, people couldn't go work. People lost their jobs. They had family members who were dying that they couldn't attend funerals for … There wasn't a single person in South Australia who wasn't affected.'

When, on 22 March 2020, Stevens moved to close South Australia's borders to other states and territories, it was the first time in 100 years that this had happened. The last occasion was during the Spanish Flu pandemic. While a 'border bubble' was at times in place allowing Victorians who lived close to the South Australian border to travel into the state unrestricted, Stevens said 'it didn't matter where you drew the line, there was always going to be someone who was adversely affected'. Sometimes the rules he put in place impacted the commissioner's own family: his son couldn't have an 18th birthday party, a close friend's funeral was restricted to a small group, and his daughter's wedding was cancelled, twice. On one of those occasions, in December 2020, he was giving a radio interview explaining why gatherings would be limited to 30. 'I hadn't told my daughter the wedding wasn't going ahead, [and] my future son-in-law heard it on the radio.'

Stevens said when he rang the premier in March 2020 to inform him of his decision to make an emergency declaration, he also told him that his first step was going to be to close the borders to the other states and territories. This proved to be a massive logistical challenge. There are dozens of entry points into South Australia. Hundreds of police were initially deployed to the major roads, and then in the next few weeks they started to close down the minor routes. But there were still farm tracks and small rural roads that they couldn't justify sending officers to, and people got inventive in their attempts to breach the border. Four young men who stowed away on a freight train to escape Melbourne's lockdown were caught in Adelaide, on route to Perth. A 65-year-old woman narrowly avoided prison time after hiding in the back of a truck to dodge a rule that for a time meant even South Australian residents couldn't return home from Covid-affected states unless their travel was deemed essential. A trio from New South Wales was arrested at a karaoke night in Coober Pedy in June 2021 after flying into the South Australian outback town on a small plane.

Another person navigating the South Australian border restrictions was federal politician Mark Butler, who would serve as Labor's shadow health spokesperson for part of the pandemic. Even as most interstate travel was curtailed, a select group of politicians still had to make their way to Canberra so the government could pass urgent pandemic-related legislation. 'It was all very weird,' Butler said. He and other MPs would fly to Canberra on air force planes, leaving and arriving out of deserted airports. Parliament House was eerily empty. No visitors were allowed. When he went back to Adelaide, Butler had to quarantine at home for 14 days. On one occasion, he remembers coming out of his two-week isolation in the morning, only to go straight to the airport to Canberra, where he spent 24 hours, before heading back to Adelaide to start a new 14-day quarantine period.

Along with real power, both the South Australian police commissioner and the chief public health officer were given symbolic prominence by the premier—a hangover perhaps from Marshall's time in business, when he might have had responsibility for the overarching operations, but the day-to-day management was left to a team. Marshall explained to another journalist, Roy Eccleston, in May 2020, that it was a deliberate strategy not to take the lead communicating to the public. 'A lot of political types said, "I can't believe when you had your 14 days with no outbreak that you didn't [announce it]," he was quoted as saying. '"Other politicians would have had the confetti cannons going off and a big announcement, and you let Nicola Spurrier do it." And I said, "Well, that's right. From day one, we all knew our role in the team."... You know, politicians have a standard format ... We didn't want that ... We wanted high-level public education, communication ...'

Spurrier became the butt of jokes in 2021 when she advised football fans attending an AFL game at Adelaide Oval, against a team from Melbourne who had been granted an exemption to get into the state, to 'duck' if the ball came near them. But at home, 'Saint Nicola', as she was sometimes nicknamed, was very much liked by the public, along with the commissioner, who gave people straight answers to their questions. Journalist Andrew Hough said it also meant that when there was the need for lockdowns and other major restrictions, the public 'went along with it', because they trusted and respected the senior bureaucrats.

Spurrier told us she was given advice early on from the chief executive of South Australia's health department, Dr Chris McGowan, that authorities needed to maintain community confidence. She said she relished the opportunity to speak at press conferences and explain things simply to people, also keeping them abreast of the overall plan. 'If things are divisive, you've lost it,' she said.

The strategy was admirable, and it seemed to work from a public health perspective. Almost everyone we spoke to about South

Australia's response described the population using the same word: 'compliant'. But where it left Marshall politically was another question. 'There was sort of a running joke that he was the sort of MC of the Covid press conferences,' Hough said. 'Towards the later part of 2021, the Labor opposition then exploited and very ruthlessly highlighted what they claimed was no political leadership, saying, "Where is Steven Marshall? What is he doing? Why isn't he making the decisions?"'

Despite the Marshall government's success in keeping Covid-19 out of South Australia, it lost the March 2022 election after one term of government. The victory by the Labor opposition, led by 41-year-old Peter Malinauskas, who famously bared what media reports described as his 'chiselled abs' at a campaign appearance at the Adelaide Aquatic Centre, was decisive. It also ran counter to the national trend in state elections in Tasmania, Queensland, and Western Australia, where success in managing the pandemic seemed to guarantee another term in government. The police commissioner said he believes Marshall didn't get the credit for the leadership he provided through the pandemic because 'South Australians saw me as the decision-maker'.

If the election had been held in 2021, the result might have been different. Marshall was punished by voters for disruptions that followed when the borders were reopened in late 2021 — days before Omicron, a new strain of Covid, was declared 'a variant of concern'. Testing centres were swamped, with waits extending to nine hours or more. Business owners were angry as people were again asked to work from home. Over Christmas, hundreds of people were forced into isolation, and a nightclub had to close after a 19-year-old partied after testing positive for Covid-19. The young man, who in the middle of the saga was probably the most unpopular person in Adelaide, was seen kissing at least two women, sharing cigarettes with friends, and hugging people, according to witnesses.

On Boxing Day, as a record 774 daily Covid cases were recorded, fresh restrictions were announced, including limited home gatherings of ten people, down from 30, and tougher hospitality density limits. Marshall names this part of the pandemic as the most challenging. 'It was devastating for many people … We were back to … restrictions on home gatherings and other restrictions which were really punishing in the lead-up to Christmas, New Year's, and the holiday period.'

South Australia actually came within a whisker of shutting the borders again less than two weeks after the state lifted its hard borders to New South Wales, Victoria, the ACT, and the rest of the world on 23 November 2021. Reporter Andrew Hough was driving his daughter to netball about 15 minutes before his newspaper's deadline on a Friday night, 3 December, when he received a call from 'a senior person' in government confirming a story Hough had been chasing for hours that day with multiple sources.

'My daughter answered and put me on speaker phone,' he said. 'The person proceeded to tell me that a decision has been made that borders were going to be re-shut.' Hough said he was told that there was to be another meeting first thing on Saturday morning, when it would be signed off, but that it was a 'done deal'. He made an eleventh-hour call to his editor, and they changed the words that had already been laid out on the front page, ready to be sent to the printers. The new version of the story said: 'South Australia's Covid-19 chiefs will today consider an emergency border lockout of New South Wales and Victoria amid rising fears over the Omicron variant.' Soon after, the article was published online.

Hough was still at his daughter's netball game when his phone started lighting up. And his phone wasn't the only one ringing. According to Hough's account, so was the police commissioner's, the premier's, the chief public health officer's, and that of the head of the Department of Premier and Cabinet. On the other end of the phone were senior business leaders, and state and federal politicians, shocked, angry, and in disbelief that the borders might close again. Hough was gardening on the Saturday morning, listening to the Covid-19 press conference, when he realised that things weren't going as he'd been told they would. 'They'd changed their minds,' he said.

Police commissioner Grant Stevens confirmed that he had seriously considered closing the borders again, but ultimately decided against it, taking account of the public sentiment. 'Part of the thinking was Omicron is so easily transmissible,' he said. 'There was a realisation that we were holding off the inevitable. Omicron was coming in because of its transmissibility, and we thought best that we bring it in and manage it, as opposed to try and hold it off, and then be caught off guard because it had snuck in and we weren't ready for it.'

South Australia's tough border rules often meant a lot of pain for the minority so that the majority could enjoy a relatively unimpeded existence. Marshall was still acutely aware of the costs carried by those locked out or disadvantaged, and of the missed funerals and the postponed weddings. 'People across the border say South Australia got away from this largely unscathed—that is not true,' he said. 'There was widespread family dislocation, work dislocation, and many businesses were very significantly affected, especially in the CBD.' While the experience of South Australians was a world away from the protracted lockdowns in Melbourne and Sydney, those measures were very much front of mind for the state's decision-makers. 'Go hard and go early was really our mantra,' Marshall said.

At the same time that New South Wales was being overrun by the Delta coronavirus variant in July 2021, South Australia managed to extinguish its own outbreak of the infectious and deadly variant through a seven-day statewide lockdown. The lockdown was announced after just five cases were detected. This time, people were allowed to exercise, but only for 90 minutes a day, and only 2.5 kilometres from home. 'If we had left it three or five days, it would have just taken so much longer to stamp it out,' Marshall said. 'Even those very short lockdowns that we had were very harsh on individuals, businesses, and families. Ultimately, that sacrifice was much less than what it would have been if we were in prolonged state lockdowns like they were in New South Wales, Canberra, and Victoria.'

In 2021, South Australia reported the strongest economic growth of any state in Australia, expanding by 3.9 per cent, compared to New South Wales, which grew by 1.4 per cent, and Victoria, which saw a contraction. South Australia has long suffered from a 'brain drain' of young people moving elsewhere in search of bigger cities and opportunities. For the first time in 30 years, more Australians were moving to South Australia than away from it. The police commissioner said it didn't escape his notice that when he was watching the morning television programs during the pandemic, it was very much focused on the east coast of Australia. 'I'd put that down to us being the quiet achievers.'

CHAPTER TWELVE

New South Wales' gold standard

It was nearing closing time at a Mexican restaurant in Sydney's eastern suburbs when a takeaway order arrived with a ping. At first glance, there was nothing particularly unusual about the meal request: a small vegetarian burrito with tofu, mild salsa, pinto beans, cheese, and sour cream. But there, in smaller writing at the very bottom of the order, were the special instructions. They contained a message from one of Australia's most experienced public health physicians, Dr Craig Dalton. There had been a Covid-19 exposure at the restaurant, Dalton warned. He urged the recipient to call him immediately. 'I don't really want a burrito, but I couldn't get through on your phone,' he added.

The date was 26 June 2021, and Greater Sydney was just hours into its first sweeping lockdown in more than a year. Every hour that was lost or gained in the contact tracing process could be critical. If this outbreak of the infectious Delta strain was unable to be contained, it would likely spill out to other states, and spell an end to Australia's Covid-zero era. For many hours, Dalton had been trying to contact the venue, part of a popular fast-food chain, but his calls were ringing out. He had tried other restaurants belonging to the same company. They were not picking up either. Then he realised that everyone ordering food from the venue must have been using an online food delivery app.

'I'm a vegetarian, so I ordered a vegetarian burrito,' he explained. 'I thought, if this gets made, I didn't want it to kill an animal.' The last-ditch ploy worked. Dalton received a call about half an hour later from a sceptical restaurant worker, and then later from several other confused people in management wanting to find out why on earth he had sent such an important message via a burrito order.

Through the first 18 months of the pandemic, the methods used by New South Wales' contact tracing teams tracking down those with Covid, and anyone they had come in contact with, seemed closer to what you might expect in a police investigation than anything else. Bank records were cross checked, mobile phone travel history was downloaded, hours of CCTV vision was examined, and potential cases were messaged on Instagram and Facebook. It is perhaps no surprise that by the end of 2020, New South Wales was being held up for its 'gold standard' coronavirus management. This reputation, seeded by the meticulous investigations of the state's contact tracing teams, blossomed in contrast to the apparent failings of its southern neighbour, Victoria.

In the winter and spring of Covid's first year, Victoria had been in its grim and lonely battle with the virus. New South Wales, led by Liberal premier Gladys Berejiklian, was able to continue to quarantine tens of thousands of returned overseas travellers and to manage a steady drizzle of cases without having to ask nearly as much of its citizens, or to put powerful business interests offside. This was no better illustrated than by the management of the coronavirus outbreak in the Northern Beaches in Sydney—an enclave of brilliant beaches and stupendously expensive real estate—at the end of the first year of the pandemic. About 275,000 residents from Spits Bridge to Palm Beach were issued with stay-at-home orders on the same day that a worrying 23 new cases were recorded. The iconic Sydney-to-Hobart yacht race was cancelled for the first time in its history. But Berejiklian rejected advice from anxious outsiders to go further and to lock down Sydney entirely.

'We held our nerve and only shut down suburbs, we didn't even go beyond those suburbs,' Berejiklian told the *Australian Financial Review*'s political editor, Phillip Coorey, in a magazine cover story boldly titled 'The woman who saved Australia'. 'I remember getting abused by other states at the time because we weren't reacting quickly enough, we should shut down the state, and why weren't we doing all of that?' she said.

Western Australian premier Mark McGowan accused New South Wales of a 'whack-a-mole' response to the outbreak, which soon saw cases spread to Victoria. Australian Medical Association vice-president Dr Chris Moy said at the time that the New South Wales government was playing the odds by relying heavily on the state's much-vaunted contact tracing system instead of imposing a quick lockdown to stop cases seeding across Sydney. 'They have put themselves and put the rest of the country at risk,' Moy told *The Age* newspaper on the first day of 2021, as the nation's hard-fought control of the virus seemed to teeter in the balance.

But the gamble paid off, as the outbreak was eventually reined in without a city-wide lockdown, as was the related cluster in Victoria, and the Northern Beaches' lockdown was lifted a week later. Berejiklian's approach kept her popular with her electorate, even after her secret relationship with a disgraced colleague, Daryl Maguire, was exposed. The claim that New South Wales was the 'gold standard' was repeated so many times that those who bestowed the accolade became blind to the vulnerabilities of Australia's largest city. Ben Fordham, Sydney's top-rating breakfast radio host, said that, for a long time, the hottest topic in Sydney was Melbourne. '[We were saying] "Oh my God, look what's happening in Melbourne, what a shitshow." And there was a degree of ridicule to it as well. '"Look how hopeless they are. Look what they are doing to the people. They are locked up forever. They are not allowed to do anything." Little did we know that the same was coming for us—it was just going to be a little bit later.'

To best understand how the pandemic was managed in Australia, you need to know who held the levers of power at different moments. Sometimes, that was a politician or an official signing new rules into law, or removing them. Other times, it was another person or persons entirely. For many months, New South Wales' daily coronavirus press conference, held at 11.00 am, was unmissable viewing for the state's residents. Berejiklian would stride out first, announcing the latest case numbers, any new restrictions, and the details of people who had died in the preceding 24 hours. 'All three were unvaccinated, a male in his 30s, a male in his 60s and a male in his 80s,' said Berejiklian in one of the briefings in late August 2021. 'Again, we extend our deepest condolences.' Most days, she was accompanied by the state's chief health officer, Dr Kerry Chant. The hard-working physician would take the public through the outbreak data in more detail.

Health minister Brad Hazzard was also there, standing behind Berejiklian and in front of a white media screen dotted with the red waratah logo of the New South Wales government. The former science teacher and solicitor had spent nearly two decades in parliament, and was nearing the end of his career, when he was faced with nightmarish projections of deaths and hospitalisations in Australia's most populous state. It was Hazzard's signature on the public health orders that imposed restrictions on the New South Wales public, unprecedented in living memory. And in the early months of 2020, it appeared that Hazzard was indeed the driving force behind the new rules. But as time wore on, and the public health orders became more universal and restrictive, the big calls were coming from Berejiklian.

Kate Aubusson, *The Sydney Morning Herald*'s health editor, said the decision-making became so centralised with Berejiklian that even the lowliest request for information from the health department had to be ticked off by the premier's office, as they sought to control the message. Berejiklian fronted the media six days a week, taking only Sundays off, for months on end. 'The public were really grateful, it seemed, that she was making the hard decisions to keep them safe,' Aubusson said.

For the first year and a half of the pandemic, New South Wales authorities were able to hold coronavirus at bay in a way that appeared easy from a distance. The state's contact tracers were held up as heroes, their real titles replaced in the media with catchy fake ones, such as 'virus detectives'. But as praise was heaped on them from outside, media interviews with the contact tracers themselves were rare. The group tried to resist becoming the face of the state's coronavirus response. They were also protective of the confidentiality of their work, which relied entirely on continued public trust and compliance. Now many of those working in senior roles in the New South Wales health ministry have revealed to us what went on behind the scenes.

Just before Covid-19 was discovered, epidemiologist Jennie Musto had returned to New South Wales from Bangladesh, where she had been on a long-term assignment with the World Health Organisation in the world's largest refugee camp, managing measles and cholera outbreaks. Musto would join New South Wales Health as operations manager for the state's Public Health Emergency Operations Centre. She said she thought that control of Covid-19 had already been lost in March 2020 when authorities were alerted to cases from the Ruby Princess cruise ship. A handful of detected infections quickly turned into several dozen. Musto remembers Chant declaring that they should 'call them all'—meaning that they needed to get in touch with every single passenger. 'That was the first time we'd ever done something like call 3,000 people.'

Contact tracing work in New South Wales had been traditionally conducted out of the state's local health districts. These established units, staffed by those with knowledge of the communities they worked in, were seen as the state's 'secret weapon' and were later replicated in Victoria. In the case of the Ruby Princess, the response was run out of the Ministry of Health's offices in St Leonards. At first, the health ministry and the local health districts were largely able to cope with the help of their own staff and those with related expertise, such as contact tracers from the Department of Primary

Industries, who usually tracked outbreaks in racehorses and other animals. As demand grew, though, the net widened. Qantas pilots, Taronga Zoo staff, and dog handlers were among those recruited to the military-style campaign.

There were just six people working in Musto's team when they received notification of the positive cases that had come off the Ruby Princess. They were able to gather another six helpers. Then a call went out for anyone else in the ministry building who was available to pick up a phone to help track down the more than 2,600 other passengers, who were now close contacts. 'We still didn't know a lot about the infectiousness of Covid at that point, but I didn't think we were going to contain it,' Musto said. Police officers were dispatched to people's houses. Letters were posted. They were sending people messages on Instagram and Facebook. Contact tracing, joked Musto, 'can be a little bit stalky'. She wonders if the older demographic of the passengers was her team's lucky break, enabling them to contain the outbreak. 'They probably don't have very large social groups, and most of them were just going home.'

If coronavirus hit Victoria like an earthquake in 2020, in New South Wales it was more like a tremor. The first cases arrived in the state on 25 January, detected in three men who had recently arrived from China. Outbreaks in March and May in Dorothy Henderson Lodge and Newmarch House, claiming two dozen lives, underscored the vulnerability of aged-care homes to a virus that was exponentially more dangerous the older you were. A steady stream of infected people flying in from overseas piled on top of cases from the Ruby Princess outbreak, before the figures tapered off as a result of the national border closure and a state shutdown. New South Wales' first lockdown, which was imposed at the same time as similar restrictions were put in place across the nation, lasted from late March to early May 2020. Restaurants and gyms were closed, public gatherings of more than two people were largely banned, and weddings were limited to a guest list of three. By 11 May, when no cases were recorded for the first time since February, the state's first wave had slowed to a trickle.

This initial outbreak was marked by a high number of infections caught overseas, which turned into a cluster of dozens of small introductions, rather than a single large one. Close to 60 per cent of the 3,095 cases detected in New South Wales between January and May had flown into the country. The last person sick from coronavirus was discharged from the state's intensive-care ward in early June, when most of the cases being reported each day were from inside hotel quarantine.

Berejiklian had resisted closing New South Wales' borders early in 2020, arguing that it was in the national interest for them to remain open. It was consistent with her approach to avoid lockdowns, border closures, and other draconian measures wherever possible. When she finally decided to close the border to Victoria on 8 July, as cases mounted there, it was reluctantly. It was the first time the border had been closed in a century. However, unknown to authorities, the disease had already infiltrated New South Wales. An infected Melbourne man who worked for a forklift company had been at a party with his workmates at the Crossroads Hotel in the outer south-west of Sydney, and had unwittingly spread Covid-19 to staff and a large number of patrons who'd dined at the bistro on the same Friday night.

'They were all sitting in this little atrium area, which was quite small and quite enclosed, and that's where the transmission occurred,' Musto explained. 'From there, it just took off.'

Berejiklian said it wasn't possible for the state to pursue a Covid-elimination strategy, as its population was too large. This meant that from July to November that year, the state recorded coronavirus cases most days—sometimes up to dozen or more. 'Every time we have an outbreak, we can't afford to lock down, reopen, lock down, reopen,' she told ABC's 7.30 program. 'That's no way to live or to be able to instil confidence to businesses to keep employing people.'

Jennie Musto, to her acute embarrassment, was publicly praised by Hazzard and Berejiklian for her work connecting the two initial cases that emerged in early July back to the busy night at the Crossroads Hotel, and was dubbed in the media as New South Wales' 'chief virus detective'. It was an important discovery, though, because it brought investigators to the index case, and flushed out hundreds of other close contacts.

Not disclosed at the time were some other breakthroughs made as contact tracers worked not just to detect cases in the community, but also to understand how infections were connected.

There was a particularly puzzling case in 2020 where investigators couldn't understand the link between two apparently unrelated cases in the same office building. Had they grabbed a coffee at the same place? Perhaps they shared lunch together? Was there transmission in the kitchenette? Eventually, the local health unit staff cracked it: the workers were having an affair, one of several uncovered during this time. Another time, the operators at a café were so desperate not to have their staff quarantined that they sent faked CCTV footage of the interaction between what they claimed was the positive case and their staff. It showed the 'infected customer' theatrically leaping back after they'd paid for their food, keeping well away from the counter as they waited for their order. The contact tracing team politely thanked them for the footage, and explained that they knew it wasn't the person in question, as they were wearing different clothes.

Craig Dalton, who was heavily involved in contact tracing out of the Hunter New England Local Health District, said it was extraordinary how many people couldn't provide accurate accounts of their movements. He estimated that one-third of recollected dates, times, and locations were so inaccurate as to be useless, or worse. Misinformation could result in hundreds of people wrongly being asked to isolate for 14 days, which made the contract tracers' work to carefully cross-check information vitally important.

A huge amount of work was also done with the major grocery

chains to try to prevent coronavirus from shutting down the giant food-distribution centres in western Sydney. Coles has a chilled distribution centre in Eastern Creek with a refrigerator that is more than seven soccer fields in size. 'It has the whole of New South Wales' food for one week in it at any one time,' said Stephen Corbett, then a director at the Nepean Blue Mountains Local Health District. 'So if it went down because of a few cases of Covid, the food supply was threatened.' Through the work of the public health officials, definitions about what length of time and type of interactions constituted a close contact to a coronavirus case were developed. Corbett said supermarket chains changed the way they allowed staff at the distribution centres to interact, to avoid a huge number of staff becoming forced into isolation.

The explanation most often relied upon to explain New South Wales' 'gold-standard' coronavirus response through the first phase of Australia's pandemic was its 15 local health districts, established in the 1990s. In a piece in *The Conversation* asking where 'did Victoria go so wrong with contact tracing?', Deakin University's epidemiology chair, Professor Catherine Bennett, argued that the decentralised units gave New South Wales an advantage. 'They're already linked with local area health providers for testing, they already have relationships with community members and community leaders, and they know the physical layout of the area,' she wrote. 'In Victoria, a legacy of cuts left the Department of Health and Human Services under-resourced and highly centralised, meaning there was a smaller base upon which to build the surge contact tracing capacity.' Victoria also had to rely on a much shallower pool of experienced public health experts when the pandemic struck. Hospital doctors were called in to run contact tracing units and to help navigate the state out of lockdown. By contrast, if New South Wales' chief health officer, Kerry Chant, would have had to step down, there were probably a dozen or more people capable of taking on her job.

Still, many senior New South Wales health officials, including Chant, hated the term 'gold standard'. Aubusson said the chief health officer never wanted the public to feel like they could rely on contact tracing alone. 'It's something that never gets quoted because it's not sexy, but she always stressed the public are partners in trying to control the spread of Covid,' she said.

The concept of New South Wales as the gold standard was born in Canberra and grew wings in political press conferences. It was first mentioned by prime minister Scott Morrison in late August 2020, and was repeated many times after, when it was often used more as a weapon to shame others than as a compliment. The inference was that New South Wales had succeeded, whereas Victoria, which remained in lockdown in the spring of 2020, was a victim of its many failings. 'New South Wales — I mean, that is a state that has built its testing, tracing, and outbreak capability to deal with shocks to the system and keep its economy open,' Morrison said when he addressed the Canberra press gallery on 21 August, flanked by two Australian flags, with another pinned on his lapel. 'I think they have set … the gold standard on how that works. They are the state which, frankly, has been under the most pressure of any state and territory in the Commonwealth. And their results today are simply magnificent.'

In a 2023 interview with us, Morrison said his approach to managing the pandemic was much more aligned with the New South Wales strategy; in his words, to only do as much as you had to. 'Ultimately, no one got everything right in the pandemic, but in Australia, we got it right more often than anywhere in the world,' he said. However, Morrison's public support for the Berejiklian government's approach was often in contrast to their reportedly frosty private personal relationship. Berejiklian allegedly described Morrison as a 'complete psycho' and as a 'horrible, horrible person' in leaked text messages made public in 2022. Morrison said because he had known Berejiklian for decades, the pair were able to have 'difficult conversations'.

'So I'm not saying we didn't have [them], we did, you think we should, we certainly did about schools, but I thought I had a honest relationship with Gladys,' he said. 'You have got to appreciate that everyone was working under incredible stress, and so people would get upset from time to time.'

Australian Capital Territory chief minister Andrew Barr said that Morrison's default position was generally not to support strict public health measures. 'It was not his instinct,' he said. Barr said what played out publicly—that New South Wales was the gold standard and that states should be able to manage things without lockdowns—also played out in national cabinet.

One of the enduring mysteries of the pandemic in New South Wales is the source of the outbreak in Sydney's Northern Beaches in late 2020. A bus driver who transported international air crew to their hotels was among the first cases discovered around 17 December that year. It seemed like they were the obvious patient zero. That case, however, was deemed to be unrelated, a diversion of sorts. Wild speculation filled the void. A false yet surprisingly specific rumour spread, claiming that Australian actor Bryan Brown and his director wife, Rachel Ward, had caught Covid in America and spread it to a personal trainer at a private session in their Avalon home. A bamboozled Brown told Sydney's *The Daily Telegraph* that he hadn't been out of the country for almost two years, did not have Covid or a personal trainer, and no longer lived on the Northern Beaches. 'I'm not on social media, so I didn't know anything about it until suddenly I was getting phone calls from everyone,' he said. 'I have no idea how it happened.'

Jennie Musto said contact tracers suspected the index case was a flight attendant who had returned from overseas and lived in the Northern Beaches, but they were never able to prove it. They traced back every single case associated with the cluster, examining CCTV footage to try to find the missing link. They pulled the records of every airline staff member who had been exempted from hotel quarantine, or others who had been given ministerial exemptions, to no avail.

The outbreak took off at two roaring gatherings that turned into super-spreading events—one at the Avalon Bowlo, a bowling club and live-music venue, and the other at the Avalon Beach RSL Club—which were held a few days apart.

It had been the first weekend since the start of the pandemic that dancing was allowed at New South Wales pubs and clubs. A local band, The Starwoods, appeared at the Bowlo to a full house on Sunday afternoon, 13 December. 'We were having a great time,' the band leader, whose stage name was Max Pistols, told *The Sydney Morning Herald*. 'We had no idea that we were walking into a cesspool.'

Within days, there were dozens of cases associated with the outbreak. Shortly before Christmas, stay-at-home orders were introduced for residents of the beaches. Some rules were also extended for the rest of Sydney. People could only have ten people at their home, but up to 300 patrons were still allowed to attend pubs and clubs, as long as they abided by density limits and other rules.

Aubusson, a long-term health and science reporter, said it became particularly clear to her at this point that the decisions on restrictions were being led by the premier's office. Almost all Sydney's super-spreading events to date had occurred in pubs and clubs. It was perplexing to her and others that they remained open. The journalist said the message she received from experts in epidemiology and infection control who worked with Kerry Chant and her team was that the officials never wanted those places to remain open, serving alcohol. 'The conclusion from these people was that this was a politically driven move. And, of course, New South Wales is famous for its pubs, liquor lobby, and its pokies, so it doesn't take a genius to see there was a lot of tension when it came to these decisions.'

Because of its tolerance for managing a low number of coronavirus cases in the community, New South Wales was often on the wrong end of border closures, meaning its residents or visitors often couldn't leave the state. From the first weeks of the pandemic, Ben Fordham's Sydney radio show started receiving many messages from people harshly impacted by restrictions. A three-year-old boy named Memphis from Queensland was separated from his parents for about two months in 2021 after going to visit his grandparents at their cattle station near Griffith in south-west New South Wales before the border closed. After the case was taken up by Fordham, Queensland Health granted the toddler an exemption to fly home. His reunion with his mother, Dominique, was captured on camera. The little boy, wearing a red shirt and little boots, ran across the airport tarmac, arms outstretched, and jumped into her arms. Sobbing could be heard in the background.

'It got to the point where we had Queensland Health on speed dial, and there would be an audible groan when they realised it was the 2GB Breakfast show calling,' Fordham said. 'Then in the end, they were going, "Righto, what's the name? What's the case number?" ... What was happening was there were so many requests coming into health departments on compassionate grounds, they admitted to us that they just weren't reading them all. They couldn't. There were tens of thousands of them. So they would just send an automatic reply to say, "I'm sorry, your request has been rejected."'

Fordham said many New South Wales residents felt genuine hatred towards Queensland premier Annastacia Palaszczuk and Western Australia's Mark McGowan for shutting them out of their states.

'It's not a word I use often, but that is the best way to describe it. It was hatred. Hatred of Annastacia Palaszczuk, a hatred of Mark McGowan, and probably ridicule of Daniel Andrews,' he said. 'There wasn't the level of hatred towards Daniel Andrews from New South Wales because none of us wanted to go to Melbourne anyway, but Sydneysiders took great delight in ridiculing him and all of these failures to do with coronavirus, even though, as time would tell, we would have plenty of them in our own front yard, too.'

Tensions around interstate borders only intensified when a new outbreak began in Sydney in June 2021, leaving thousands of Victorians trapped in New South Wales, some effectively homeless, or paying double rent, or having no income. Before the borders closed in July 2021, farmer Jose Garcia drove eight hours down the Hume

Highway from his property in Lancefield in Victoria to the rural town of Oberon, on the western fringe of the Greater Blue Mountains in New South Wales, to visit his elderly parents. His father was in the final stages of dementia and living in an aged-care home, while his mother was booked in for joint surgery, following years of chronic knee and hip pain. But when Garcia's father died suddenly the day before Garcia's permit to return to Victoria expired, the 56-year-old extended his trip to be with his grief-stricken mother. His wife, Sonya, who was stuck on the other side of the border looking after the family farm on her own, and his daughter, were unable to come to the funeral.

When Garcia made an application to get home to Victoria, the permits were meant to be processed within a fortnight, but two weeks came and went with no word from the government. Finally, an email landed in Garcia's inbox. 'It said words to the effect we've closed your case. If you still want to come to Victoria, then reapply,' he said. Garcia frantically filled out another application, but weeks passed again with no word from the government. He tried to call countless times. Each time, he would speak to a different staff member in a call centre. He said one operator even blamed him for this situation. 'They said you were given plenty of warning. Why didn't you just go home weeks ago? I tried to tell them my father has just died and I need to get home to my family,' he said. 'I've never been somebody who has needed counselling or anything like that. But you sort of think to yourself, am I ever going to get home?'

It would be three months before Garcia was finally allowed back into Victoria, and only after he had provided the Victorian government with a copy of his father's death certificate. Garcia was so distressed by the experience that he packed up his home in Victoria and moved to Queensland in late 2022.

What struck Victorian ombudsman Deborah Glass most about the management of Victoria's border closures to New South Wales was 'the absolute heartlessness of it all'. The lawyer said Victoria's border regime resulted in some of the most questionable decisions she had seen in her career. 'When we began looking at this, I thought we would find an overstretched system that just collapsed under the weight of all of these requests coming in for exemption,' Glass said. 'I was shocked, because what we actually found was a system that was putting an enormous amount of effort into keeping people out.'

There were 315 complaints about the scheme to the ombudsman, including from people unable to access urgent medical care, and from a woman who left Victoria to help her daughter with her premature twins, only to be barred from returning home to tend to her flock of sheep, which had no food. In another case, a woman was asked by officials why she could not put her intellectually disabled sister in aged care while she was unable to be her carer. Between 9 July and 14 September, 2,649 applications were made to attend a funeral or to be with a dying loved one. Only 877 were granted. Another 10,812 requests were made on health and compassionate grounds, with only 895 granted. Glass said decisions to keep Victorians out of their home state were not being made by low-level officials who were just overwhelmed by applications. Instead, she said the decisions were being made by senior health bureaucrats and officials in the health department who were effectively looking for ways to say no and to block people from entering Victoria.

'The amount of effort that was going into preventing them from getting in was mind-blowing,' Glass said. 'There was this absolute lack of nuance and compassion that had its origins in what appeared to be a culture of caution within the Victorian Department of Health. Everybody felt that if they made a decision that allowed somebody in and that was going to seed an outbreak, that they would be blamed or be the one responsible for allowing them in.'

Amanda Garner's daughter Harriette, who attended the Yanco Agricultural boarding school on a rural New South Wales farm, was left stranded and unable to get back to her family's farm in Birregurra in Victoria's south-west, when the state snapped its border shut. Harriette was boarding in a remote part of New South Wales where there were no detected coronavirus cases. The Victorian government wanted Harriette to fly to Sydney, the epicentre of the outbreak, and then fly back to Melbourne, which was being engulfed by another coronavirus wave, and to spend two weeks in hotel quarantine. Garner was so distraught that she almost moved across the Victorian border just to be with Harriette, who had been separated from her identical twin sister, Milly. 'We were so focused on getting the twins back together again,' Garner said. 'They were missing each other terribly.'

Harriette was one of ten Victorian boarding school students stuck in New South Wales. Garner and some of the other parents whose children were trapped on the other side of the border considered sneaking across and smuggling their children home in the back of a cattle truck in the middle of the night. 'It was brutal,' Garner said. 'It felt like eternity before we saw her again.' It took almost a month for Harriette to get home to Victoria, where she did a two-week stint in a quarantine hotel in Melbourne with her father, Richard, before being reunited with her mother and twin sister.

'It was just crazy. No, she's not a baby. But they were verbalising that my child was a risk to the Victorian population,' Garner said. When the family's case was reported in the media, Garner recalls people on social media calling her a 'selfish pig' for wanting her daughter home with her. 'People were dying, and there was so much fear about the virus,' Garner said. 'It divided people, and tore some families apart for a time.'

CHAPTER THIRTEEN

Queensland's border wars and the great migration

The night the 'Great Wall of Coolangatta' first went up at the New South Wales and Queensland border, Lauren Blong and her family were roused by flashing lights and the 'beep, beep' sound of reversing vehicles. Blong, who owned a homewares store called Sparrow and Fox on the New South Wales side, about 30 metres from where the two states meet, was temporarily living with her family in the space above her retail shop. With her two children in tow, they walked outside and headed towards the commotion. They found trucks, loaded up with bollards, and police and state emergency services personnel in orange uniforms, setting up a checkpoint next to a motel and roundabout near the centre of town.

The border line that separates the coastal towns of Coolangatta in Queensland and Tweed Heads in New South Wales was usually invisible, lost between the palm trees and high-rise motels. It was common for people to have medical appointments on one side and to take their children to school on the other. But during the pandemic, dystopian images emerged from the border zone. Father's Day in 2021 saw separated families gathered in large numbers on both sides of the long orange barrier snaking along the suburban street that marked state lines. Police wandered slowly along each side, dispensing face masks.

The border was closed for the first time on 5 August 2020, as New South Wales reported cases linked to a funeral gathering, and as Queensland approached a state election. It would stay sealed for 250 days. When the virulent Delta strain emerged in 2021, the border was set up again between 22 July and 13 December. Queensland Premier Annastacia Palaszczuk declared, 'We're putting Queenslanders first.' But for many of those whose lives and livelihoods straddled the Queensland and New South Wales border, it wasn't that simple. Some people were eligible for a pass that allowed them to cross into Queensland, and yet there were still cases of healthcare workers and medical administration staff unable to travel between the states to work, and reports of business owners sleeping in their stores instead of their homes on the other side of the border.

The second level of the Blongs' store had been casually sub-leased to tarot readers and healers, but those tenants had moved out when much of Australia's non-essential industry was shut down in March 2020. This meant that the Blongs had to pay the rent for several retail spaces and their family's unit, without having any clear idea of how they would make enough money to cover the bills. So they moved into the shop secretly. They showered at their friend's gym nearby, which had also been closed, and they stayed quiet every night as a security guard did his rounds, jiggling the locks. The kids thought it was a great adventure.

Blong said there were many border jumpers. Some people had a car on both sides, and just hopped over the barrier and jumped into their other vehicle. 'You could walk over, for ages,' she remembered. 'You could walk over, you could ride your bike over, you could roller skate over, but as soon as you were in a car, or a motorbike, you had to have a border pass.'

In the end, the orange bollards that had been set up to physically divide a community became the place where people came together. The fence became a table, cluttered with food to share and takeaway coffees. Some set up fold-up chairs. Children and babies were passed over. There was a constant stream of people walking past the Blongs' store, sometimes carrying picnic gear, and sometimes a gazebo, to the orange wall. 'We'd go take packages up to that border and hand them to customers who couldn't come over. It was quite communal.'

Tweed Heads shire councillor and president of the town's chamber of commerce, Warren Polglase, remembered people jumping in dinghies early in the morning before the sun rose, and sneaking off to work in Queensland. He said the pandemic measures were brutal on small businesses, and that some never recovered. Tradespeople would bring tools and timber, and drop them at the border for their colleagues working on projects in Queensland. Polglase celebrated his 80th birthday party at the border. His family came from Queensland, and they popped bottles of champagne and ate prawns together. 'It was certainly a memorable birthday,' he said.

Queensland Premier Annastacia Palaszczuk's office is deep inside Brisbane's historic Parliament House, where political decisions have been thrashed out since the late 1800s. The Renaissance revival-style building is surrounded by manicured, lush lawns and gardens. A row of ferns beneath Palaszczuk's office became the backdrop to the regular Covid-19 press conferences led by the premier, Australia's longest-serving female head of government.

Our interview with Palaszczuk occurred on a characteristically sunny and muggy day in Queensland. Palaszczuk was wearing an emerald-green shirt and pearl earrings, and was quick to offer a cup of tea and a plate of colourful macaroons. The conversation quickly turned to the days of the pandemic in Queensland. Palaszczuk recalled barely sleeping at the time. 'It was very stressful,' she said. 'You're just waking up [in the middle of the night] thinking, *Have we done everything here? What more can we do?*' At the forefront of her mind was Queensland's ageing population. 'This was life-and-death scenarios with projections of tens of thousands killed from the virus and, of course, it was going to have a big impact on seniors,' she said. 'We were absolutely determined to protect our seniors at all costs.'

Queensland's hardline health approach and early action, led by its then chief health officer, Jeannette Young, a doctor who thrives in the fast-paced world of emergency medicine, was lauded globally for the lives it saved. Their Covid-zero approach meant that people lived who would otherwise have died. Mass outbreaks were quickly contained or avoided entirely. Lockdowns—of which there were only a handful—lasted days, not weeks. As Victoria and New South Wales were sent into consecutive lockdowns, the great migration began. More than 107,000 Australians from all over the county relocated to warmer climes in the subtropical sunshine state, known for its pristine beaches and Great Barrier Reef, in search of a relatively Covid-free existence.

The pandemic caused significant disruptions to all major sports in Australia, but, in the words of sport studies lecturer Steve Georgakis, perhaps the most fascinating, and unlikely, was the 2020 AFL grand final being played in Brisbane. Queensland beat off competitive bids from South Australia and Western Australia to secure the rights to host the event at the Gabba (the Brisbane Cricket Ground) on 24 October. It was the first time in history that the match was played outside Victoria. The grand final is a sacred day for many Victorians, but that year the game between Richmond and Geelong was played under lights at night, to avoid a clash with the Cox Plate horse race in Melbourne and the heat of Queensland's late-afternoon sun. The state's borders had been closed to Victorians, meaning that the only viable route to the grand final was via the Northern Territory and a mandatory fortnight's quarantine at an unused workers' village in Darwin's rural outskirts. Footy-mad Victorians forked out $2,500 to quarantine in Darwin just to attend the game, which Richmond won by 31 points.

Queensland's tough stance on keeping its borders shut to states that were being ravaged by coronavirus was a point of political contention. To some, Queensland's closed borders embodied their safety. To others it was brutal and lacked compassion, separating families when loved ones were dying or when funerals were being held. Dozens of Australians were left stuck at the edge of New South Wales, waiting for exemptions to cross the border. Like displaced refugees, they lived in camping areas in tents and caravans. By the end of 2021, there were reports of 11,000 stranded Queenslanders, including a backlog of nearly 3,000 applications for exemptions with Queensland Health, and more than 8,000 applications for border passes with Queensland Police. For those in the tourism and business sectors, this led to economic disruption. The state's approach would spark a bitter dispute between Palaszczuk and prime minister Scott Morrison. Shots would also be fired by neighbouring premier Gladys Berejiklian as tensions escalated between Queensland and New South Wales. It became known as the 'border wars'.

In the early months of the pandemic, there was a strong sense of cooperation between the states and territories and the federal government. 'Everyone wanted to do the best for their state and their country,' Palaszczuk reflected. 'There was a real sense of unity.' Morrison had set up the national cabinet, and it was embraced by all premiers as a genuine effort at national coordination. 'The very way we interact with each other must change, and it must change today,' Palaszczuk said at a press conference on 18 March 2020. 'Our lives and the lives of our loved ones depend on it. This is a deadly virus, make no mistake, and it is here in Australia. We are in the fight of our lives.'

But as the pandemic rolled on, some states grew increasingly unhappy with Canberra. Resentments brewed about the sluggishness of the vaccine rollout, or about continual coronavirus leaks out of hotels used to quarantine returned travellers. No premier was more vocal about their grievances with the federal government than Palaszczuk, who frequently went head-to-head with Morrison.

'There were lots of instances when there were some pretty strong attacks coming out of the federal government,' Palaszczuk said. 'When it all broke down, it felt very personal. The consequences of that are still there to an extent today, and it just didn't need to be like that.' Palaszczuk said she holds the former prime minister and his public criticism of Queensland's handling of pandemic restrictions responsible for some of the many death threats she received during the pandemic. She also revealed the frustration she often felt when Morrison sought out advice from male premiers, describing a boys' club culture that often excluded her.

'I think he liked speaking to the men and not to the women,' Palaszczuk said. 'I would be interested to find out what Gladys's [Berejiklian's] recollection of that was. But often he referred to conversations he'd had with Dan [Andrews] or Mark [McGowan] or Steven [Marshall] or the boys, rather than myself. But it doesn't matter, you just get on and do the job.'

Palaszczuk worked around the clock, and for almost two years her life was transformed into a rush of press conferences and meetings. 'I have a very close family, and at times I couldn't see them, so that was difficult,' she said. 'We all learnt to zoom, and we all learnt how we can stay connected.'

A simmering backlash about the impracticality of the border between New South Wales and Queensland led to Palaszczuk attempting to shift the checkpoint from Coolangatta to the Tweed River, to allow Tweed Heads residents to cross seamlessly into Queensland, but Berejiklian rejected the idea. 'Unfortunately, the New South Wales premier wouldn't support that proposal,' Palaszczuk said. 'It would have solved a lot of issues over those areas, because there are schools, there are hospitals, and people share those community facilities around those areas.'

Palaszczuk and Berejiklian had vastly different ways of dealing with the Covid-19 pandemic, observed Queensland political journalist Lydia Lynch. Both leaders assured their communities that decisions were underpinned by health advice, she said, but Palaszczuk was cautious when lifting restrictions, while Berejiklian imposed less tough restrictions in the hope of keeping the economy ticking along. Their public digs at each often made headlines. Berejiklian criticised Palaszczuk many times over the border closures, describing them as 'ridiculous' and costing people their jobs. The Queensland premier was quick to fire back: 'We are not going to be lectured to by a state that has the highest number of cases in Australia,' she said.

There were gritted teeth and verbal jabs between the pair when either was questioned about the other at press conferences. A series of text messages were leaked to *The Daily Telegraph* revealing that Palaszczuk had taken three days to respond to a message sent by Berejiklian congratulating her on her party's Queensland election victory in 2020. When Palaszczuk did respond, all she wrote was one word: 'Queenslander' after the Maroons' win over the New South Wales Blues in the rugby league state-of-origin game. After details of the texts were leaked, Berejiklian later told reporters she 'didn't know whether to be shocked or bemused'.

But, despite the friction between the duo, Palaszczuk said she harboured no ill feelings towards Berejiklian, adding that the media often played up the idea of a fractured relationship between the two women. In fact, she said she admired her. 'I look back on it, and Gladys was just trying to do the best for her state, and I was trying to do the best for my state,' she said. 'And, you know, I have always had respect for her. She was in a difficult situation. We were all in a difficult situation.'

Palaszczuk is far less forgiving of Morrison. During the federal election campaign in 2022, in a scathing rebuke of his handling of the pandemic, she suggested that Morrison had missed a 'golden opportunity' to unite the nation. Morrison hurled barbs back, accusing the Queensland premier of 'extortion and holding the government to ransom' when she had demanded more hospital funding before she would reopen the state's borders in 2021. Then, in another stoush, Palaszczuk stood in a windswept field outside Toowoomba and declared that her government would go it alone and build a cabin-based quarantine facility without any Commonwealth cooperation. But perhaps no attack would sting the Queensland government more than the case of Sarah Caisip, who wrote a letter about not being allowed to see her dying father in September 2020:

Dear Premier, my dad is dead and you made me fight to see him, but it was too late, and now you won't let me go to his funeral, or see my devastated 11 year old sister. You are preventing me (a 26-year-old woman) from going to view his body, which is a very important tradition for me, and also preventing me from going to his funeral this Thursday. I came from virus-free Canberra, so the fact that I'm even in quarantine is beyond belief but the fact that I am being denied my basic human rights to care for my grief-stricken mother and little 11-year-old sister enrages, disgusts and devastates me at the same time.

The family's anguish gained national attention after the letter, shared on Facebook, caught the eye of Morrison. He went on radio station 2GB in Sydney, declaring he had personally appealed to Palaszczuk to overrule the decision. 'It's not about borders, it's not about Federation, it's not about politicians, it's not about elections,' Morrison said. Caisip, a nurse in Canberra, had initially been denied an exemption to leave hotel quarantine to say goodbye, despite arriving from the Australian Capital Territory, where there were no active cases. There was a tense public stand-off between Morrison and Palaszczuk, whose government compromised and allowed Caisip a few minutes alone with her father's body at the end of the funeral.

When questioned about the matter in parliament, Palaszczuk went on the attack, labelling the raising of the matter as 'disgusting'. 'I will not be bullied, and nor will I be intimidated by the prime minister of this country,' she said, adding that while it was a tragedy for the family, the decision was the chief health officer's to make. Palaszczuk faced a slew of attacks and a surge in death threats in the aftermath, as people accused the state of a 'cold-hearted' border regime. Days after Morrison publicised the case on radio, a banner was flown over Brisbane and the Gold Coast with the words 'She is heartless' scrawled across it. Caisip's family would later accuse Morrison of politicising their family's tragedy.

When asked later about his relationship with the Queensland premier, Morrison described the tension with Palaszczuk over the Caisip case as 'regrettable and very unfortunate', adding that he had never intended for it to blow up the way it did. Morrison said that Palaszczuk, whom he had not known as well before the pandemic as some other premiers, and whom he had a limited rapport with, had been 'very supportive' of him and the national cabinet early on, describing her as a premier who 'pulled no punches'. But he acknowledged that when you are from two different sides of politics, it can be easy to damage trust.

The director of infectious diseases at Mater Health Services in Brisbane, Associate Professor Paul Griffin, has praised Queensland's swift action at the beginning of the pandemic. He said that the closed borders undoubtedly protected Queenslanders and saved thousands of lives before vaccines arrived. However, he believes that Queensland became a victim of its early success. 'I can completely understand why we did want to limit people's movements across the borders at certain points in time,' Griffin said. 'But we had a response that was one of two extremes. It was a little too harsh early on, and it lacked common sense and compassion around some of the rules. But then we became perhaps a little too liberal.'

Griffin is an infectious disease physician who works in several Brisbane hospitals. He is acutely aware of the dangers of allowing a highly infectious disease such as Covid-19 to run rampant, and throughout the pandemic was a staunch and vocal supporter of lockdowns before vaccines were rolled out. However, Griffin said there were several instances in the first two years of the pandemic when Australians needed urgent medical care in Queensland, but potentially life-saving treatment was unacceptably delayed or missed out on due to the border closures.

'I was certainly involved in some cases where there were people who were essentially not able to enter who needed medical services that really were only feasibly available in south-east Queensland,' Griffin said. 'We had always provided those services, and suddenly these people can't get into the state.' Palaszczuk sparked a national outcry in August 2020 after her government refused entry to a woman from New South Wales requiring medical treatment, declaring, 'In Queensland, we have Queensland hospitals for our people.'

Griffin said he and his colleagues repeatedly raised concerns to the government about delays in people receiving care between the borders, and the difficulties that healthcare workers and patients were experiencing in obtaining exemptions. 'In certain parts of northern New South Wales, for example, there were very unwell babies who then had to go to Sydney, rather than coming to south-east Queensland, which was a lot closer for them. That's when I think it went a little bit too far,' Griffin said.

The senior physician said that he was personally distressed by families not being able to come into Queensland to be with their dying relatives. 'I feel very strongly that compassion was something that should have been part of the response, and not allowing people to see their dying relatives is not something that you get a chance to do over,' Griffin said. 'Very early on, we knew enough about how to control the risk, and we could have allowed people, within reason, with some reasonable precautions, to visit their dying relatives. A good-quality N95 face mask, for example, when worn properly, can go a very long way to protecting people.'

Palaszczuk said that Queensland's border policies were always reflective of the best health advice at the time. 'Looking back on it, I do appreciate how difficult that was at that time, when we were so used to being able to go to the airport, travel around, hop on a bus, get in a car, and we were basically telling people, no, you have to stay at home, and during that time people did pass away and had a big impact,' she said. 'I do acknowledge all of that.'

Chief health officer Jeannette Young faced intense online trolling and death threats over decisions that led to people not being able to attend funerals and see their dying loved ones. During a heated press conference in September 2021, she clashed with reporters over the continuing Queensland and New South Wales border dispute, vowing that interstate borders would not open until 'every single person in the state' had been offered a vaccine. When asked by reporters how many deaths she would be comfortable with in order to get to 'Covid normal', Young appeared frazzled and at the end of her tether before she snapped.

'Come on? Can you please remember who I am? I stand up here every day, I went into medicine to save lives. I'm not comfortable with any deaths that are preventable, so that's why I want every single Queenslander to get vaccinated, because that is the best protection.'

Young strongly defended the border closures publicly, maintaining that she 'always made it very, very clear that anyone who urgently needed care, of course, they could immediately come to Queensland'. In January 2021, her extraordinary influence over Queensland's Covid-19 response was the subject of a parliamentary inquiry, which examined if too much power had been granted to her. 'I do not exercise these powers lightly,' Young told the inquiry. 'These measures do infringe people's liberties, but only to the extent necessary to ensure we do not let this virus spread into the community.'

Asked what pandemic moments stand out most to her, Palaszczuk recounts a visit to Cherbourg, an Aboriginal settlement in Queensland in late November 2021. Concerned about lagging vaccine rates among Aboriginal people in Queensland, Palaszczuk spent the day going door-to-door with local health groups providing Covid-19 vaccinations to Aboriginal families in their homes. 'We saw some evidence that showed that if the virus got into some of our Indigenous communities, it could be devastating,' Palaszczuk said. 'We were very keen to increase vaccine rates, and to try everything we could.' Palaszczuk also highlighted the Indooroopilly State High School cluster, where 137 infections were linked to an outbreak, including 60 students and five teachers across five schools, plunging 15,000 people into home quarantine for two weeks. It had all the hallmarks of a superspreading event, but disaster was averted by the community efforts, which Palaszczuk said summed up the Queensland spirit. 'Everybody just did the right thing around that whole area,' she said. 'It should have been spreading everywhere, and we actually contained it and stopped the spread. People really stepped up.' Palaszczuk said the astronomical surge of migration to Queensland was a reflection of the state's extraordinary success in suppressing the virus.

Andria Cozza was part of the great migration, fleeing Melbourne in April 2021 and settling in Burleigh Heads, nestled between glistening Surfers Paradise and laidback Coolangatta. 'It has a really nice energy about it, and it's just a beautiful community,' Cozza said. 'I felt really connected to the place, almost like I had lived there before.' The 38-year-old had been craving a change for years, but the catalyst for uprooting her life was Melbourne's protracted lockdowns.

In early 2020, Cozza had felt elated during a trip to Brazil, where she spent months learning Samba and Afro-Brazilian dance. She then paraded with a Samba dance school at the Rio Carnival, a tradition dating back to the 17th century, which has become synonymous with the cultural identity of the South American country. Each day, Cozza was surrounded by hordes of sweaty people who took to the streets to party in one of the world's greatest displays of escapist hedonism. There were lots of glitter, feather boas, sequins, and scantily clad dancers swaying to the beat of drums. Social distancing was an unheard-of concept.

She remembers frantically packing her suitcases and rushing to the airport in Brazil as it was announced that Australia's borders were snapping shut, and arriving home the next day to an apocalyptic lockdown in Melbourne. 'Brazil was magic,' Cozza said. 'Coming back to Melbourne was like coming home to a huge vortex. You're thinking, *What is going on? Is this even real?*' Cozza's hopes of further establishing her career as an early-childhood teacher were dashed by continuing lockdowns, which disrupted employment opportunities. She described living alone during the lockdowns as 'lonely and horrendous'.

Before the pandemic, she could never have imagined leaving her close-knit Italian family and friends behind in Melbourne. But she took the plunge, and has thrived. 'It is so interesting, because every second person is from Melbourne here,' Cozza joked. 'They all say they just had to get out of Melbourne. It was like this mass exodus.'

Victoria's overall population plummeted by almost 50,000 to less than 6.6 million during the pandemic. Queensland was the go-to state for Victorians, with 23,299 moving north through 2020 and 2021.

Queensland's lockdowns were minor blips compared to those that Melbourne and later Sydney experienced. The state's first brush with coronavirus was on 21 January 2020, when a man who had returned from Wuhan in China was the first person in Queensland to record a positive test result. The state government declared a public health emergency. Queensland entered its first lockdown on 23 March, and within a week had reported almost 700 cases of coronavirus. Travel outside the home was banned except for essential reasons, and restrictions did not start to ease until 2 May.

The next lockdown did not occur until 8 January 2021, prompted by the infection of a hotel quarantine cleaner who had caught the virus and spent five days in the community. This lockdown was lifted three days later, although millions of residents were asked to continue wearing masks in indoor public places for a further two weeks.

At the end of March 2021, Greater Brisbane was ordered into a third snap three-day lockdown, in response to a cluster of infections linked to the Princess Alexandra Hospital. Its fourth lockdown was enforced on 29 June 2021, when several cases, including a 19-year-old casual receptionist at the Prince Charles Hospital in Brisbane who had travelled to Magnetic Island and Townsville, were found to have been in the community while infectious.

In late July 2021, south-east Queensland went into a snap lockdown until 8 August, after six infections with the Delta variant were detected. But just as south-east Queenslanders emerged from lockdown, Cairns residents were plunged into a snap three-day lockdown of their own after a local taxi driver was found to have been infectious in the community for ten days with coronavirus.

By July 2021, only seven Queenslanders had succumbed to the virus. Its fatality rate in the first 18 months of the pandemic was just under one death per million residents—the lowest rate not just in Australia, but in any sizable jurisdiction with its own policing and health powers in the world. Queensland had reported only 2,000 infections by December 2021, compared to 136,000 in Victoria and 86,000 in New South Wales.

'I'm very proud of Queensland's record,' Palaszczuk said, adding that she is still stopped on the street by Queenslanders who thank her for having kept them safe. 'People are really beautiful and kind. They still come up and say thank you for looking after us.' When Palaszczuk made history on 31 October 2020 by becoming the first female premier to win three state elections, it was considered a reward for her handling of Covid. Traditionally blue-ribbon conservative seats, such as Caloundra on the Sunshine Coast, switched to Labor for the first time in history. In her victory speech, she thanked the 'many people' who had voted Labor for the first time, including the so-called 'Palaszczuk pensioners'.

And the Blongs' gift store, which had seemed so under threat during the Queensland and New South Wales border wars, is now thriving. Making a virtue of necessity, the Blongs spent time during lockdown, when they weren't permitted to open their shop, in building an online business, finding a global market for their crystals and other wares. By the third year of the pandemic, they had gone from a team of two to a staff of seven. They were no longer living above the store.

CHAPTER FOURTEEN

Patient zero

The television reporter held up her microphone to the intercom of a modest block of yellow-brick flats in Sydney, and asked accusingly: 'Do you take any responsibility for this outbreak?' At the other end of the line was the man by then best known to Australians as 'the Bondi limo driver'. His name was Michael Podgoetsky, the suspected 'patient zero' in a Covid outbreak that was about to shut down Sydney and then send many millions more Australians into lockdown. It is thought he caught a dangerous variant of the virus when transporting a three-person FedEx air crew from Sydney Airport. With Podgoetsky sick at home, and his wife, Elina, briefly hospitalised, reporters had been ringing his intercom again and again. 'I'm coughing. My head aches. Then there's the intercom, pressed non-stop from seven o'clock till the night,' he told us.

The Azerbaijan-born grandfather was cast as the villain after his infection was confirmed by a nose and throat swab on Wednesday 16 June 2021. A police investigation was swiftly launched into his conduct and whether he had complied with public health orders. Yet Podgoetsky also had many of the hallmarks of those who have most often been the victims of the coronavirus pandemic: a migrant, vulnerable to misinformation, and a small-time contractor without access to sick leave. Like many thousands of Australians, he was fearful of the AstraZeneca vaccine, believing that his history of blood clots would put him at higher risk of the rare side effect. Elina Podgoetsky said she had rung New South Wales Health seeking a Pfizer vaccination for her husband and herself in May, but had been refused as they weren't eligible.

As well, New South Wales' public health orders hadn't required Podgoetsky and other international airport drivers to be vaccinated or to wear a mask. At this stage of the pandemic, vaccines still provided considerable protection from Covid-19. (Later variants would be much better at evading vaccine-acquired immunity.) Former senior public servant Jane Halton, who in 2020 had conducted a review of Australia's hotel quarantine arrangements, was horrified by this turn of events. She had reportedly already identified the transport arrangements for international crew as a 'potential hole' in the quarantine system, and warned the federal government about this.

As the Bondi outbreak began to take hold, New South Wales premier Gladys Berejiklian was asked why these frontline workers weren't subject to mandatory vaccinations. 'I'm as upset and frustrated as anybody,' she said. 'We all worked so hard, and it's really disappointing when things don't go the way they should.' Omar Khorshid, the president of the Australian Medical Association at the time, argued that the virus leak was a failure of government 'in a way worse' than the bungles associated with the Victorian hotel breaches that had led to the state's second wave because, by this time, so much more was known about Covid and how it spread. 'It was just unfathomable that he wasn't required to be wearing a mask, and … everyone involved in hotel quarantine should have been at the absolute top of the list for vaccination … It's just a no-brainer.'

While it was widely reported as fact that Podgoetsky was not wearing a mask when driving infected transport workers, the Bondi resident of more than 40 years insists that he was wearing one.

Some of the memories from this time still haunt the Podgoetskys, and have lost none of their sting. One of those occasions was when Elina Podgoetsky, who caught Covid around the same time as her husband, was discharged from hospital and was taken to hotel quarantine for three nights so she could be monitored. Podgoetsky said that all she had with her was the clothes she had been wearing: tights, a T-shirt, and a puffer jacket, plus her handbag. Because her daughter was also in isolation, she said there was no one who could bring her supplies to the hotel. She said nurses who visited the hotel to check her oxygen levels told her they had only scrubs to give her, and call-takers on the New South Wales Health line weren't able to help, either. That left Elina with no pyjamas. 'I was so cold, because you know during Covid, you're really shivering … I had to wrap myself in a towel and put my clothes from the hospital in the washing machine and dryer, and then for the next two days I had to wear the same clothes because I was so cold I didn't want to wash them again. It was an awful, awful, awful experience. I will never forget that in my life.'

The couple also described a series of encounters they had with reporters. There was one television journalist who climbed the steps to their apartment and knocked on the front door when the Podgoetskys were still in quarantine and probably still infectious. 'She was banging our door, saying, "Michael, are you there?"' recalled Elina Podgoetsky. 'Imagine if we would have opened the door? She will get sick.'

Another, they said, followed them across town to a medical appointment, and then remarked that he didn't have much time if he was going to file his story for the six o'clock news.

More than a month after police had decided there was insufficient evidence to charge Podgoetsky with any breaches of the law, a reporter from *The Daily Telegraph* found him sitting at a bus stop near his house without a mask on, in violation of the strict rules at the time. The newspaper promptly sent photographs of him to the police. His full name and his picture were plastered on the front page of the Sydney tabloid. 'Limo driver unmasked,' blared the headline, highlighted in red. 'He's the limousine driver dubbed the "index case" in the nation's worst Covid outbreak—and the law has caught up with him,' the story read. Podgoetsky said he had been wearing a mask that morning as he left his apartment, but had taken it off because his glasses had started fogging up and he had a 'spinning head'.

'I decided to sit down at the front of my home on the bus stop,' he said. 'I'm cleaning my glasses and also ordering Uber, because I need to pick up my car from Bondi Junction Service.' Police were waiting for him when he arrived home in the afternoon, and he was fined $500.

The Podgoetskys insist that the experience hasn't changed the way they feel about Australia—'the best country on earth'—but the words of those who shamed and blamed them still ring in their ears. 'Imagine that everybody thinks that you're responsible for a lot of deaths in New South Wales and then maybe in Australia,' said Michael Podgoetsky. 'It's just a horrible, horrible weight to carry on your shoulders.'

The emerging Sydney Covid cluster was handled in the same way that New South Wales had generally approached its other outbreaks, relying on its lauded contact tracers to do the heavy lifting. Prime minister Scott Morrison appeared on the breakfast television show *Sunrise* about a week after Podgoetsky tested positive. He commended premier Berejiklian for 'resisting going into a full lockdown', and said he was 'very confident in the ability of the New South Wales government, which they've demonstrated time and again dealing with these situations'.

But this outbreak was not the same as the others. The Delta strain that had entered the country was estimated to be about twice as infectious as the original Wuhan-variety Covid. The federal government was so concerned about the Delta variant's capacity to breach Australia's quarantine system that, the month before, they had controversially ordered a temporary ban on travellers from India, where the strain had first been detected. This had left more than

9,000 Australians stranded, while hundreds of thousands of Indians died.

'India is burning, and the Australian government doesn't seem to understand that it is a war zone here,' Melbourne man Bhaumik Dholakiya said in May 2021. His father died in the outbreak. 'There are dead bodies being burned on the streets. We understand the need to protect Australia from this virus. It is a country we love, and it is our home. But we are feeling alone and in great distress.'

Dholakiya was stranded in India for weeks while his entire family was infected and the country's hospitals ran out of beds and oxygen, leaving people to die in lines waiting to see doctors. After a fierce backlash and accusations of racism, Morrison announced soon after that the ban would be lifted and that repatriation flights would resume.

The cases trickled in slowly at first, one or two a day. Initial exposure sites included cafés in cliffside Vaucluse, department stores in busy Bondi, and a Sunday cinema screening of *Hitman's Wife's Bodyguard*. On a day that 10 new cases were announced, face masks were made mandatory in public indoor spaces in Greater Sydney, the Blue Mountains, Wollongong, and Shellharbour. The next day, a further 16 cases were detected, and people in Sydney and surrounding areas were told that they could only have five people in their home. Drinking standing up at a pub was banned (although sitting was permitted). Dance floors were closed, except for the bridal party at weddings.

Senior public health officials who were leading the response to what was known as the Bondi outbreak were growing increasingly concerned, and they began agitating for a lockdown. Three senior New South Wales Health officials told us that advice was given to the government to take stronger action in the face of the unfurling outbreak, but it wasn't taken. As the restrictions were slowly ratcheted up, the experts argued it was happening too slowly. Craig Dalton, the eminent physician who was involved in contact tracing in New South Wales and also helped in Victoria in 2020, said he was most concerned that the daily case count was being treated as a real-time measure of the outbreak, when in reality those numbers lagged a week or more behind the actual transmission incidents. 'I would say myself and 90 per of my colleagues wanted much earlier interventions,' he told us. 'We just knew that we couldn't possibly be capturing all the cases.'

Jennie Musto, the operations manager for New South Wales Health's Public Health Emergency Operations Centre, also confirmed that she was part of the group pushing for an earlier lockdown. She said that officials didn't give written advice when they knew it was not going to be accepted, but 'it was given'.

Stephen Corbett, who was at the time a director at the Western Sydney and Nepean and Blue Mountains local health districts, said that there was general agreement among the public health unit directors that the interventions were not going far enough. 'Measures such as closures of schools and workplaces had massive impacts on the economy and the financial hardship being endured by the community. Unsurprisingly, there was strong political opposition to some of these,' Corbett said 'Kerry Chant and other public health leaders were in the unenviable position of having to make recommendations about effective measures with information that was far from perfect.'

Chant was known to seek counsel widely, having regular and long conversations with an extended inner circle of experienced epidemiologists and public experts, floating ideas or getting their opinion on their particular area of expertise. She sought out those who she knew were likely to have a different opinion from her. Professor Allen Cheng said at times he was speaking to Chant daily. Epidemiologist Professor John Kaldor would also receive regular calls from the New South Wales chief health officer. He described her approach as pragmatic. There were times in the pandemic he would suggest that she try a certain thing, and although she wouldn't say it explicitly, it was clear that she knew the idea wouldn't be politically acceptable. 'She would always say in an indirect way that she's got to do what's feasible.'

Chant wasn't a public figure before the pandemic hit and doesn't welcome the spotlight, rejecting most interview requests that come her way. On the few occasions she has submitted to a personal profile, she has given little away and is more comfortable talking about the achievements of her team rather than herself. Kaldor sees her as a future director of an Australian centre for disease control, and has told her as much. 'In my opinion, she's far and away the most competent and experienced public health official in this country,' Kaldor said.

Greg Hunt, the federal health minister, told us that senior federal government health officials were trying to help Chant lobby the New South Wales government to be 'more aggressive in their steps' to contain the Delta outbreak—citing resistance, not from Berejiklian, but from members of her cabinet. He said federal treasurer Josh Frydenberg also was in touch with Dominic Perrottet, the New South Wales treasurer, about financial support that the federal government could put in place. In a taste of his attitude to coronavirus restrictions, Perrottet was reported to have suggested during the Northern Beaches outbreak that Chant take a pay cut of 5 per cent if Sydney suburbs were unnecessarily locked down. The suggestion was that Chant, a bureaucrat, might not fully comprehend the consequences of a business shutdown on ordinary people.

Hunt's impression was that there was a view within the New South Wales government that they had stared down the outbreaks in 2020 and the preceding summer, and that they could do it again. But it was Hunt's opinion that the 'borders, testing, tracing' strategy that had worked earlier would not be enough for Delta. 'Their tracing system was vastly superior to Victoria's, but Delta was just a completely different animal … [it] meant you had to have restrictions on top of the other three elements to contain it.'

On Saturday afternoon on 26 June 2021, a press conference was hastily called following a crisis meeting of the New South Wales cabinet. Gladys Berejiklian strode out to the microphone, peeling off a blue surgical mask. 'Are you guys okay?' she asked, swivelling around to quickly address Chant and Hazzard, who stood behind her. A look of distress flitted across her face. The day before, stay-at-home orders had been issued for residents living in four areas of eastern Sydney. Now, with 29 new cases having been detected, many of them people who had been out and about while infectious, the lockdown was now being extended to the whole of Greater Sydney, including the Blue Mountains, the Central Coast, Wollongong, and Shellharbour. The 4.8 million people living in those areas could only leave home for four 'essential' reasons: shopping for basics; for compassionate needs or medical care; for exercise in groups of ten or fewer; and for work and education, where it was not possible to work or study at home.

'The New South Wales government has always prided itself on taking the expert health advice,' Berejiklian said in her opening remarks. 'And even though we don't want to impose burdens unless we absolutely have to, unfortunately this is a situation where we absolutely have to.'

The plan was for the lockdown to last only two weeks, but epidemiologist and World Health Organisation adviser Professor Mary-Louise McLaws was quick to hose down expectations of a short shutdown. 'The horse has bolted, but the horse started bolting last week,' she said, telling us at the time that her home state would be 'lucky' if the lockdown only lasted a fortnight. The popular media talent, diagnosed with brain cancer soon after, said that a shutdown should have occurred just days into the outbreak. That would have prevented a birthday party in the western Sydney suburb of West Hoxton being held on Saturday 19 June, which led to 24 of the 30 people who attended becoming infected. (The only people who didn't catch Covid were vaccinated.) The party wasn't a 'super-spreading event', she argued. It was just the contagious Delta variant behaving normally.

Morrison had publicly cheered on New South Wales in its approach to Delta in the critical early days of the outbreak, and had probably done the most to cultivate the idea of New South Wales setting the gold standard for how to manage Covid outbreaks. But as the state continued to break daily records for new cases, and as people began dying, he changed his position. 'It's important to note that early and stringent and short lockdowns will be necessary to deal with outbreaks in this Delta strain,' he said in late July the same year. 'That is a clear learning of the events of recent weeks and months in terms of the activity of the Delta strain and the work we have looked at around the world to inform that decision.'

When asked by a journalist if he regretted 'applauding premier Berejiklian for resisting a full lockdown last month when case numbers were rising,' he claimed that people were acting on the advice that they had and the information they had. 'No one in the world has perfect hindsight over these issues. The Delta strain is a strain that we've sought to understand and learn [from], and react to and respond to. So those who have had to make those decisions have made decisions, I think, in the best interests of their state and on the best possible advice they had available to them. I'm in no different situation to that.'

In late August, news broke that a 30-year-old mother of three had died with Covid at her home in Sydney's west. The state's virus death toll stood at 132.

When Delta struck, it was no longer possible for the New South Wales contact tracers to engage in the same level of detective work that they had applied in previous outbreaks. They were working unsustainably long hours, and were scrambling to find new staff to help. Associate Professor Kate McBride, an epidemiologist who was seconded from Western Sydney University to help with training new staff, estimates that there were fewer than 20 contact tracers working at Western Sydney public health unit when the first cases emerged, and that 'a huge shortfall became apparent almost immediately'. McBride said at times they were so stressed that they almost felt numb to the confronting things they were being exposed to.

One day, she was trying to track down a patient, concerned that he might have not been isolating, or was in hospital. She finally discovered that his body was at the morgue, and she started laughing, in shock. 'It's just like, *Oh, I found him, he's dead*,' McBride recalled. 'It was really bad.' They were often having to issue section 62s to force people with coronavirus who didn't believe in the virus, or were refusing to isolate, into special health accommodation. 'We had absconders, young guys who would go to work, and you'd be trying to find them in a grocery shop in western Sydney.'

While McBride believes the Delta outbreak would have been uncontainable even if they had had a 1,000-strong contact tracing team, she said some of the surge workers lacked a crucial under-standing of the local community, a place where it was not unusual for people to live in multi-generational households of ten people or more. She said that although she loved working with the teams from the defence force (she joked that her swearing worsened by the day), for some of them, 'there was little understanding of context, and a lot of laughing about names'. McBride said the need for a bigger reserve workforce of contact tracers remained a big topic of conversation, and that she would like to see all public health workers trained in the skill.

Although Covid was rapidly brought under control in the affluent Sydney suburbs where it began, it quickly established itself in the most disadvantaged areas of the city, across town in south-west and western Sydney. In these places, roughly 38 per cent of the popula-tion speak a language other than English, a figure that swells to 90 per cent in some suburbs. People here would be infected more, die in much higher numbers, and have greater restrictions placed on their freedoms.

Even though harsh restrictions targeting specific postcodes in Melbourne had failed to bring Victoria's second wave to heel, a similar strategy was applied in Sydney. For many weeks, if you lived in one of the nominated council areas in the sprawling west or south-west, you were not allowed to leave your neighbourhood unless you were an essential worker. You had to wear a mask outdoors. Recreation activi-ties such as picnics were banned. Hundreds of army troops were sent to check that people with Covid were isolating and to help police set up roadblocks. A daily curfew was later introduced, spanning the eight hours from 9.00 pm to 5.00 am, for 12 local government areas that were home to two million people. These included Bayside, Blacktown, Campbelltown, Canterbury-Bankstown, Cumberland, Fairfield, Georges River, Liverpool, Parramatta, and Strathfield. None of these rules applied elsewhere in Sydney.

Kerry Chant was not happy with this approach. She recommended in an email in August 2021, released many months later, that strict lockdown rules be implemented consistently across Sydney. Chant had spent a decade as director of the public health unit in south-west Sydney, and was said to be particularly troubled by the impact of coronavirus and restrictions on this community and others like it.

While the confidentiality provisions of crisis cabinet were often used by the New South Wales government to avoid giving specific details of the health advice they were receiving, the New South Wales Audit Office confirmed in late 2022 that during the Delta outbreak, the state government 'did not always act on advice' when it came to its Covid response. The office identified several occasions where there were delays of between three and 21 days from advice being given and a relevant decision being enforced. It also confirmed that New South Wales Health was aware well before the Bondi cluster that the Delta strain was 'significantly more infectious' than predecessor variants, so much so that what had worked previously in New South Wales was likely to fail. 'New South Wales Health identified the risk that due to the local levels of vaccination, community transmission was unlikely to be controlled with Test, Trace, Isolate and Quarantine alone, and social measures such as mask wearing and density restrictions in public places would be required,' the audit office report said.

As it happened, it took two days for masks to be made mandatory on public transport in Sydney, four days for masks to become mandatory in select areas of Sydney, and a week for any social-distancing and density measures to come into force in Greater Sydney. By 3 August, Sydney's Delta outbreak had grown to close to 4,000 cases. Dina Ntaesh was at home in the kitchen when her sister-in-law called just after 2.00 pm. She remembers the sound of her sobbing into the phone.

'Your brother, he is not OK, he has collapsed, and he's not breathing.'

'Call an ambulance,' Ntaesh told her, her chest tightening with panic.

'The ambulance is already here,' was the reply. 'They are saying his heart has stopped beating.'

When Ntaesh arrived at her brother's home, she found a swarm of ambulances and police cars at the front of her brother's unit in the suburb of Warwick Farm in south-west Sydney, a neighbourhood where many dozens of the 199 Covid cases detected in New South Wales that day were clustered. Ntaesh's brother, Aude Alaskar, aged just 27, was the 17th death in the Sydney Delta outbreak. At the time, the forklift driver was the youngest person reported to die in New South Wales after contracting Covid, his death making national news headlines. The Delta strain would prove more harmful to young people: more than 13 per cent of the dead were aged in their 50s and younger, compared to less than 5 per cent during other Covid waves.

Minutes before Aude Alaskar died, his brother had spoken on the phone to the aspiring soccer player, when he had complained of a splitting headache and crippling fatigue. He promised to call straight back after he had a shower, but he collapsed in the bathroom and never regained consciousness. It was the 13th day of his isolation period. 'Time stopped moving that day. It was so horrific,' Ntaesh said. 'He was the most amazing brother. We have this empty place in our hearts, in our houses, in our lives. There is always something missing. I dream about him all the time. When I close my eyes, I see his smiling face.'

Her brother had married his wife, Yasmin, only weeks earlier.

They had met because Yasmin was a disability support worker for his mother. Yasmin later caught Covid at work, unknowingly infecting her new husband. 'He was so in love with her,' Ntaesh said. 'If she was in pain, he was in pain. Their wedding was cancelled because of coronavirus restrictions, but they couldn't wait to start their lives together, so they married in a small religious ceremony so they could always be together.'

Aude Alaskar's family are from Iraq and are part of south-west Sydney's 5,000-strong Mandaean ethno-religious community, most of whom reside in the Liverpool and Campbelltown areas. Their ancient religion can be traced back 2,000 years to Mesopotamia, an area that is now modern-day Iraq and Iran. The Mandaean community reveres John the Baptist, who they call Yehyea Yahana. Many of them, like Ntaesh's family, fled the Middle East to escape religious persecution in areas occupied by Islamic State following the rise and fall of dictator Saddam Hussein.

An outbreak during the Delta wave infected 70 people from Sydney's tight-knit Mandaean within days. Two of them died within a week of each other. Aude Alaskar's family suspect that coronavirus caused his death, but performing an autopsy goes against the Mandaean faith, which believes the body of the deceased must be pure. The pandemic would rob them of ancient customs, such as ritually washing and dressing him in white clothing, and laying his body out in the family home so each person could say goodbye.

Ntaesh, who has lived a devoutly religious life, said she lost her faith in government in the months following her brother's death. 'I felt betrayed and angry at the government for not understanding people like us, for not doing more to protect my brother,' she said. 'We still have the grief inside of us because we couldn't say goodbye to him.' Their mother remains grief-stricken. Rarely a day goes past when she does not weep for her son. She spends hours a day in quiet prayer. At his childhood home in south-west Sydney, he is immortalised: photos of him, with his warm, brown eyes and smiling face, are everywhere. His crisp, white wedding sheets are folded neatly on the bed. Ntaesh said she can still smell his aftershave in the bedroom. 'I go in there so I can still feel him with me.'

Aude Alaskar, affectionately known as 'Ady,' had been unvaccinated, at a time when Australia was grappling with a shortage of Pfizer, the vaccine recommended for younger Australians. Ntaesh is adamant that her brother was not anti-vaccination, but said he had delayed booking a vaccine appointment, expressing anxiety and fear to his family about potential side effects of the Pfizer vaccine, some of which he had heard and read about through misinformation and conspiracy theories circulating online or being spread within his community. 'His death scared so many people,' she said. 'He died, and so many people in our community and the Middle Eastern community ran and got the vaccine.'

Only days before Aude Alaskar's death, the Australian Technical Advisory Group on Immunisation issued new advice for people living in greater Sydney, urging those aged between 18 and 60 to seriously consider any available vaccine, including AstraZeneca. But by then, Alaskar was already infected. Rumours swirled after his death, fuelled by coronavirus conspiracy theorists, including social media influencer Maria Zee, who bizarrely claimed that Alaskar had never had coronavirus and that he had come back to life, but medical staff had 'destroyed the paperwork'.

Through the first years of the pandemic, people from culturally and linguistically diverse communities, or those living in poverty or disadvantage, were much more likely to die from Covid than were wealthy Australians. This was particularly striking during the Delta wave, when more than 70 per cent of people who died from Covid-19 in Australia were born overseas. Those born in the Middle East were over 23 times more likely to die from the virus than those born in Australia, and the death rate for those born in North Africa and south-eastern Europe was close to ten times higher.

Respected health economist Stephen Duckett said that Covid became a disease of disadvantage in Australia, and that there were several reasons why coronavirus death rates in Australia were highest among migrants and essential workers. 'The first is that people on lower incomes are often in more precarious or insecure employment. They're also in jobs that are more people-facing—hospitality, or aged care, or disability jobs, for example. They often have to work in multiple locations,' Duckett said. 'So you've got a situation where people of lower income, lower socio-economic status, are more exposed to risk. So it is therefore likely that, just because of that increased exposure, they're going to have more disease.'

Duckett said the effects of ageing on health are not evenly distributed throughout the population. Age-related morbidity is more common among people with less education, less money, and less access to health care. Migrant and minority groups frequently have a higher prevalence of certain health conditions, such as diabetes or high blood pressure, amplifying the risk that Covid-19 will affect them more intensely. 'Often, due to circumstances, they are unhealthier to start with, and so they're more likely to be more adversely impacted. They already have an increased risk of exposure, and if exposed, there is the double whammy of poorer health to begin with, which significantly increases risk of serious adverse outcome or death,' Duckett said.

He believes that a major failing in Australia and globally early on in the pandemic was that public-health messaging about the coronavirus and the vaccines was too often only available in English, leaving migrant communities unable to access or understand essential information. It was left to their own community leaders to repeatedly translate, to turn 'government speak into community speak,' to spread messages, and to answer questions. There was a common slogan used in Australia at the time that 'We are all in this together.' But Duckett said that those words, aimed at unifying people, to encouraging them to abide by rules and lockdowns, could not have been further from the truth.

'We are not all in this together,' he said. 'Very often, you hear this rhetoric, or you hear people referring to "hard-to-reach communities", which is a phrase I never use. The reason I never use it is because those communities can reach themselves. It is we, who are white Anglo-Saxon Australians, who are the ones saying they are hard to reach, and sort of blaming them for that. What we should be asking is why did it have to come to this? Why the hell haven't we developed the skills to actually engage with these communities, with proper health messaging and adequate support, in a systematic and ongoing way?'

Duckett said there had been a tale of two pandemics in Australia. One was merely disruptive for people who were able to pack up their desks and take work home; they emerged in the aftermath relatively stable — physically, psychologically, and financially. But the virus carved a different path through the most disadvantaged and culturally diverse suburbs. 'The ones with the least to begin with hurt the most,' Duckett said. The other pandemic devastated those who survived it, leaving lasting scars.

CHAPTER FIFTEEN

The vaccine race

They started arriving in the early evening. There were hundreds of them, clutching blankets and old plastic milk crates, braving the cold, ready to camp out under a dark winter sky. First it was mostly Sydney's Asian community, Chinese and Vietnamese families. They spilled out of hired buses driven to a vaccine clinic set up inside the Lebanese Muslim Association headquarters, a grey building with curved, tinted-green windows, next to the Lakemba Mosque in the Canterbury-Bankstown council area, which was then in the middle of a deadly coronavirus outbreak. Some slept huddled on the ground, their bodies spaced out by socially distanced orange traffic cones. By 3.00 am, the Arabic-speaking community started to arrive. They sat in fold-out chairs sipping coffee as the sun rose, hoping to secure a Pfizer dose. By dawn each morning, the line spilled beyond a kilometre.

Ahmad Malas, who was running the clinic as an organiser for the Lebanese Muslim Association, arrived every day at 5.30 am and stayed until every last Pfizer vaccine vial had been used. 'We were vaccinating about 1,500 people every three days,' said Malas. 'People began to realise that the only way out of lockdown, the only way to go back to work, was to get vaccinated. Suddenly, this little clinic we set up was cutting across all cultures, so we set up another 20 clinics.'

It was August 2021. Pfizer was scarce in Australia, but demand for it was fierce. Every day when the clinic ran out of Pfizer, there was an uproar. Hundreds of vials of the AstraZeneca vaccine were stocked in fridges inside the Lebanese Muslim Association building, but were left unused, due to fears over a rare side effect. Volunteers and doctors would make their way down the queue, urging those waiting to consider being immunised with AstraZeneca instead. But usually by then, the crowd had already erupted. Chants of 'We want Pfizer' echoed down the street. Some days, tensions boiled over, and security guards would be brought in to break up angry protests. 'It was very, very sad, because there just wasn't enough supply of Pfizer, there was a mishandling and shortage of vaccines from the government's side, but what it showed was that most people were really keen to take the vaccine,' Malas said.

Then the crazy rumours started. Malas was accused by some members of his Lebanese community, many of whom the 40-year-old had known since he was a little boy, of working in cahoots with the government and of pocketing $300 for every vaccine. The truth was that he took time off from his full-time paid job to volunteer to help with the vaccine efforts. When an older member of Sydney's Lebanese community died from unrelated medical problems shortly after getting vaccinated, the Lebanese Muslim Association was accused on social media of killing him. Carloads of people would drive past the mosque yelling out 'Sheep' and baa-ing out car windows.

'It was very distressing, because obviously people in our community were getting very sick at higher rates than anyone else in Sydney … the death rates among the Middle Eastern communities just kept climbing,' Malas said. 'There was a barrage of misinformation circling around online, and the government was pointing the finger at south-west Sydney and western Sydney. There was this sense at that time that everything was just out of control.'

Malas said that Islamic funeral parlours in Sydney's west and south-west, where the virus was spreading at breakneck speed, were struggling to keep up with rising numbers of people dying during the Delta wave. 'People from our community were being buried in double bags, which meant you couldn't perform the usual Islamic rituals, like washing and shrouding the bodies, and so people were accusing us of not following the Islamic way,' Malas said. Meanwhile, in northern and western Melbourne, an almost identical crisis was unfolding, in culturally diverse, multi-faith communities with pockets of socio-economic disadvantage and a severe shortage of general practitioners were being plagued by coronavirus infections. These were the communities that needed to be inoculated most, and yet they were also grappling with the severest shortages of vaccines in Australia.

A slow and often patchy vaccine rollout had allowed anti-vax sentiment and hesitation over being vaccinated to brew. In early September, general practitioner Umber Rind woke from a restless night, grabbed her phone, and shared a post on social media. The post, written by Rind's colleague and a fellow Muslim doctor, revealed that dozens of Victorians with coronavirus who were on ventilators in intensive-care units were unvaccinated members of her own tight-knit Arabic-speaking community in Melbourne's northern suburbs. The scenes confronting doctors were likened to a horror movie—young and old in induced comas, strapped to breathing machines, their organs failing. 'This is not an exaggeration. It is a catastrophe,' it read. 'They are our people. Not one of them is vaccinated. The numbers are stacked up against us unless we act together. Covid is real.'

To the outside world, Australia's vaccine rollout was limping along at a glacial pace. 'One day a rooster, the next a feather duster,' the United Kingdom's *Financial Times* declared in an editorial lamenting the country's vaccine rollout. 'Sydney in lockdown, borders shut and hardly anyone vaccinated. How long can Australia go on like this?' asked American news outlet CNN. A headline of an article published in *The Age* and *Sydney Morning Herald* posed a similar question: How had Australia's vaccine rollout turned into a 'train-wreck'? Countless targets in Australia's vaccine rollout were being missed in the early months. The nation, once hailed as a success story globally for its containment of coronavirus, was slipping behind the rest of the developed world with its immunisation program.

For its 'snail pace' at the beginning, the nation's coronavirus immunisation program became known as a 'strollout'—a term invented and popularised by the Australian Council of Trade Unions' boss, Sally McManus. Strollout was dubbed the word of the year by the Australian National Dictionary Centre in 2021. The centre's director, Amanda Laugesen, said that the expression captured 'a very particular moment in our nation's history'.

On the opening day of the Wimbledon tennis tournament on 28 June 2021, one of the British scientists behind the Oxford-AstraZeneca vaccine, Dame Sarah Gilbert, received a warm and sustained standing ovation from her seat in the Royal Box. In Australia, when Tennis Australia president Jayne Hrdlicka mentioned the coming vaccinations, the crowd booed.

AstraZeneca was supposed to be the backbone of Australia's vaccine program. The federal government had ordered 53 million doses, most of which would be made onshore, making it cheap and available. But frequent disruptions to the vaccine rollout and changes to clinical advice around AstraZeneca, due to the rare risk of it causing a potentially fatal blood-clotting condition, thrombosis with thrombocytopenia syndrome (commonly known as TTS), left it the poor cousin of the nation's vaccine effort. Doctors were tipping it down the sink, worried that their excess supply of doses would soon expire in fridges.

Questions were mounting about why Australia was not investing in more messenger RNA (mRNA) vaccines, such as Pfizer or Moderna, amid emerging data that they were much easier to reconfigure to cover new, more infectious variants of coronavirus than more conventional types of inoculations such as AstraZeneca. Tensions bubbled as states went head-to-head with the federal government over supply shortages. State-run clinics, including Melbourne's Royal Exhibition and Convention Centre and the Melbourne Showgrounds, were for months operating well below capacity because thousands of people avoided the life-saving AstraZeneca vaccine while they waited until more Pfizer doses arrived.

Years later, the Victorian health minister at the time, Martin Foley, remained frustrated by the way the federal government had often 'abrogated their role' during the pandemic crisis, including during the vaccine rollout, when the Commonwealth sought to publicly blame states for supply problems. 'You'd sometimes have to go on teleconferences the same week with them and just suck a lemon, because you had to ignore the fact that they were undermining you politically, and maintain the relationship to resolve this crisis,' Foley said.

It took scientists just two days to create the first Covid vaccine. In a remarkable feat of human endeavour, the first inoculations were approved within a year. In early November 2020, prime minister Scott Morrison, ddressed in a white lab coat and blue surgical mask, appeared in a laboratory in Sydney's eastern suburbs, declaring, 'Today is another day when we can look forward to a much better 2021.' The cause of his optimism was the signing of a deal for 10 million Pfizer doses, the first vaccine approved for the country. 'We aren't putting all our eggs in one basket,' he assured the public.

Four months later, on 15 February, the first batch of 142,000 vials of Pfizer arrived at Sydney airport to elation and fanfare, before being shipped to a secret location and then distributed to where they were needed most: high-risk groups, including older Australians at risk of severe disease, aged-care residents, healthcare workers, and people working in hotel quarantine and border control. Morrison famously declared that the vaccine rollout was 'not a race'. The choice of words would come back to haunt him. What happened next was a mixture of bad luck, politics, a global shortage of vaccines, missed opportunities, and poor messaging about the vaccines.

Still wounded by criticism over the early global shortages of infection-protection supplies from unreliable international supply chains, the federal government was keen to have vaccine supplies manufactured on home soil. The Commonwealth placed huge orders for homegrown supplies: a combined 85 million doses of AstraZeneca and an untested University of Queensland–developed vaccine. The University of Queensland candidate and AstraZeneca, to be produced by biotech firm CSL, would put Australia 'at the top of the queue if our medical experts give the vaccines the green light,' Morrison proclaimed proudly. But within months, both vaccines would be in trouble.

It was nine days after Professor Eddie Holmes uploaded the genomic sequence for Covid-19, in January 2020, when University of Queensland professor Paul Young received an email offering him the opportunity of a lifetime. Scientists at the university had been working on a new and unique form of technology called a 'molecular clamp', which promised to fast-track vaccine development and modification, and to offer increased protection against the inevitable new variants of coronavirus. The global vaccine-development body, the Coalition for Epidemic Preparedness Innovations, emailed the university to ask if their invention could be deployed to make a new Covid vaccine. Young and his team were ecstatic. It was the stuff scientists dream of.

They eagerly took up the challenge, and produced a vaccine candidate. As *The Age*'s Farrah Tomazin and Clay Lucas wrote in 2021, the untested technology would form half the initial backbone of Australia's entire vaccine strategy. But they were left shattered when the vaccine did not make it past phase-one trials after it turned up some false-positive HIV results, because the vaccine's signature 'clamp' technology contained an HIV protein. While this would not have given people HIV, it could have derailed Australia's HIV screening programs. 'It was absolutely devastating, because we felt like the whole country was behind us, and you feel like you've let people down,' Young said.

The team worked tirelessly for almost six weeks to try to fix the problem. Phase-one data had shown that the vaccine was safe, extremely well tolerated, and induced the hoped-for antibody response. But, following medical advice, Morrison dumped the vaccine and terminated the billion-dollar contract. 'We argued at the time there may be some value in moving to phase two or three, but the window of opportunity wasn't taken,' Young said. 'In hindsight, the right call was made. In science, nothing is ever guaranteed. There was always a risk, but when things didn't go right it was very tough.'

The next blow came when reports began to emerge from the United Kingdom and Europe in early 2021 about the AstraZeneca vaccine being linked to the very rare, but serious blood-clotting side effect known as TTS. Initially, the UK's Medicines and Healthcare Products Regulatory Agency, and its EU counterpart, the European Medicines Agency, urged their populations to keep getting inoculated with AstraZeneca as the virus raged in the Northern Hemisphere, arguing that the benefits outweighed the risks for all adults.

Back in Australia, the virus had been temporarily eradicated, and with it the urgency to be vaccinated. AstraZeneca started to get a name for being a second-rate vaccine. Early clinical trials showed that Pfizer was almost 95 per cent effective at preventing severe disease, compared to AstraZeneca's 70 per cent efficacy. Media coverage focusing heavily on the very rare complication linked to AstraZeneca did nothing to help its cause. It did not seem to matter that AstraZeneca was a life-saving vaccine, in abundant supply in Australia. Pfizer became the vaccine of choice, but there was not enough of it available. For months, accusations and questions flew about when the federal government had met with Pfizer and why they had not ordered more supply sooner.

The fiasco surrounding Pfizer and Australia's supposed bungled deal with the pharmaceutical giant was dubbed the greatest public-policy failure in Australian history. ABC journalist and co-host of the popular *Coronacast* podcast Dr Norman Swan broke the story of bad relations between Pfizer and the federal government, reporting on his podcast that three sources had told him an identical story about an inexperienced health department representative haggling rudely with

Pfizer over the cost of the vaccines and the intellectual property owner-ship. It put Swan on a collision course with the Morrison government, who vehemently disputed the accusation. Swan stood by his reporting.

The truth of the matter was never fully resolved, although documents released under freedom-of-information legislation soon after unravelled part of the mystery. The documents showed that the first discussion between Australia and Pfizer had occurred on 26 June 2020, just as coronavirus cases in Victoria were rushing upwards. Within ten days, the state would be in its second lockdown. This was followed up by a 30 June email to the health department and an attached letter to the federal health minister, Greg Hunt. The tone was direct: 'I am requesting this meeting at the earliest opportunity', the Pfizer representative wrote. The landscape was 'moving swiftly, including through engagements with other nations,' they said. In the letter to Hunt, Pfizer said it was employing its decades of scientific expertise to create a vaccine that 'could be deployed at unprece-dented speed for the prevention of COVID-19 infection'. Despite the letter being addressed to Hunt himself, only departmental first assis-tant secretary Lisa Schofield was dispatched to a meeting, *Guardian Australia* reported. A year later, both Morrison and Hunt came under fire for not having met directly with the Pfizer leadership.

The UK signed up for 30 million doses on 20 July. Two days later, the US signed a deal for 100 million doses. By November, Australia was a global outlier. It wasn't until Victoria's second wave ended that the nation finally signed a contract with Pfizer. The Commonwealth has denied that it failed to build up a broad portfolio of vaccines, arguing that, in the end, it secured five agreements that together provided more than 195 million doses. On top of the Pfizer deal, which was later increased to 40 million doses, and AstraZeneca, it also secured deals with Moderna and Novavax, meaning that the suite of vaccines was more than enough to cover the whole adult population.

From Hunt's beachside hometown of Mount Martha on Victoria's Mornington Peninsula, the retired politician said that Pfizer had told the government it was prioritising supplying countries where there were imminent deaths and 'people dying in their thousands, tens of thousands'.

Hunt said that the government had pushed for many months to get supply from Pfizer, and held 13 meetings with the company. He strongly disputed any suggestion that there were so-called secret meetings with the pharmaceutical giant, as suggested by Swan. 'There was no more Pfizer that was available in any other quantity earlier,' Hunt said. He points out that Australia received its first shipments of Pfizer in the same week as New Zealand and Japan.

'Those companies made it clear they did not have certainty of supply, and they would give us the absolute maximum they could, but it would be very limited and not until at least February of 2021,' he said. 'So we ordered everything that was available.' Hunt, keen not to focus on matters of early supply, also points out that the government vowed to get 70 per cent of the adult population vaccinated by the end of October 2021. And it did. But it was not as simple as that.

On 8 April 2021, Morrison and health minister Greg Hunt held a snap late-night press conference that some experts would later argue killed the public's confidence in AstraZeneca. Of course, this was never the intention. Morrison held the press conference to inform the public that the nation's vaccine advisory board, Australian Technical Advisory Group on Immunisation (ATAGI), had advised them that Pfizer vaccine should be given to Australians aged under 50, amid concerns of rare blood clots linked to the AstraZeneca vaccination.

The advice from ATAGI was carefully thought out and balanced. It did not preclude people under 50 from getting the AstraZeneca shot. Rather, it urged them to weigh up the risks with their doctor. In an outbreak where Pfizer supply was limited, adults younger than 50, 'should re-assess the benefits to them ... versus the rare risk of a serious side effect', the advice said. But the nuance of the risk of the rare clotting syndrome versus the huge benefit of being immunised against a deadly disease was seemingly lost in translation. The implications of this were devastating, as vulnerable older Australians began to shun the vaccine, contrary to health advice.

A former national president of the Australian Medical Association, Omar Khorshid, pinpoints this late-night press conference as the tipping point for much of the confusion around AstraZeneca and a disintegration in public confidence in the vaccine rollout. 'That press conference with Scott Morrison and Greg Hunt at night in the middle of the week, straight after they got the advice from ATAGI, was just unnecessary. All it did was scare people,' Khorshid told us over coffee on a sunny spring day in 2022, at one of his favourite cafés in Nedlands, an inner-western suburb of Perth.

While the orthopaedic surgeon believed that informing Australians of changing clinical advice related to AstraZeneca was absolutely necessary, he questioned the timing of the announcement: 'Why could they have not waited until the morning and calmly got the message out then?' In trying to be transparent with the population, Khorshid said that ATAGI had been 'unintentionally naive'.

'The way they interacted with the government was partly to blame for the hysteria in the community around AstraZeneca,' he said. 'Nobody wanted to be seen to be hiding anything. They didn't comprehend the right level of risk to explain to people in a way they could understand the risk versus the overwhelming benefit.'

When AstraZeneca's credibility took a hit, Canterbury Bankstown general practitioner Jamal Rifi said the intensity of his work in trying to convince people to be immunised more than tripled. 'People began refusing AstraZeneca, and the younger generations began to put pressure on the older generation not to be vaccinated,' Rifi said. 'The older generation, who needed the vaccine most, became afraid of it. It was the worst situation I have ever dealt with in my life, because some of these people actually passed away after refusing the vaccine. It still hurts me, because I always felt that the role of the kids is to protect their mum and dad.'

In the lead-up to the late-night press conference, ATAGI, comprising a team of 18 of Australia's most respected immunisation experts, had spent weeks analysing months of local and international safety data on AstraZeneca. Professor Allen Cheng, who was then co-chair of the vaccine advisory committee, said the group had called an urgent online meeting on 2 April 2021, Good Friday, the day after the first suspected case of the rare clotting syndrome linked to the vaccine was detected in Australia. The patient, a 44-year-old man, had been admitted to a Melbourne hospital on 1 April with blood clots in his abdomen after receiving the vaccine. Immunisation experts dialled in from all over Australia. Many were on Easter holidays or camping trips with their families. Cheng's co-chair, paediatrician Christopher Blyth, was sitting under a radio tower in the Kimberly in Western Australia, known for its large swaths of wilderness, rugged ranges, and dramatic gorges, when he called in. The realisation that AstraZeneca had been linked to a very rare but serious complication was a heart-sinking moment for all of them.

'We had this Good Friday meeting where we all discussed in detail that first case of TTS with haematologists,' Cheng said. 'Then, the following week, a second case was detected, which was also quite severe. It was then we thought, *We have to say something*. There was a lot of discussion around, well, if we are not sure, we need to say we are not sure. We need to say what we do know about this issue, because people are going to make decisions on whether or not to get vaccinated, and we need to provide them with the right information.'

The condition was caused by an immune response to the vaccine, triggering blood clots and a low platelet count, which could lead to bleeding problems. Although the condition was rare, early estimates were that it occurred in one in 100,000 vaccines. Mortality was high in the early days—the United Kingdom reported that about 25 per cent of those with TTS died. There are risks to every aspect of medicine, Cheng said, but it is one thing to sit down with a patient in a doctor's office and carefully lay out the risks and benefits of an impending surgery, and a very different matter altogether to explain the nuances of a vaccine to a population of millions of people who are understandably on edge after their lives have been upended by a deadly virus.

'We decided to have a lot of preference wording in the advice, which turned out to be a difficult message for people to hear, as it was very confusing,' the epidemiologist and infectious disease physician said. Cheng noted that in April 2021 there were almost no cases of coronavirus in Australia, so the team was weighing up the future threat of outbreaks against the current risk of vaccine side effects.

Cheng, a gently spoken and widely respected infectious disease physician, recalled the group agonising for many days over the carefully crafted words released to the public. But he conceded that once the advice was out in the wild, they lost control of the messaging. 'You don't have the opportunity to explain nuance—other people are explaining it for you,' Cheng said. 'I think that's the hardest part.'

Paediatrician Christopher Blyth, the former head of ATAGI, told us during an interview in 2021 that the advisory group had felt compelled to make the difficult call following weeks of robust debate among committee members, when it had become painfully clear that the risk level for the under-50s age group was unacceptable. 'This was not a small or whimsical decision—it was very hard,' he said. 'There is significantly more than deaths to talk about. We've got some people who have had significant medical complications from this.'

Soon after, public commentary from a number of political leaders, including Morrison, who sought to blame ATAGI for the botched rollout and to accuse them of being too conservative and risk-averse, only added to the confusion. But ATAGI had an unenviable job, trying to balance the threat posed by the virus, which was constantly changing, with the real risks of rare vaccine side effects.

In the end, the worst-case scenario forecast for the rare clotting syndrome linked to AstraZeneca did not come to fruition. Doctors became better at detecting and treating it, and it turned out to be far less common than initially feared. By October 2021, the risk of dying from TTS after a first dose had plummeted to about one in a million in people. By June 2022, there had been 88 confirmed cases of TTS in Australia, from more than 13.8 million AstraZeneca Covid-19 doses. Eleven people died from the vaccine, including eight from

TTS, during the same period. Hunt believes that the change in clinical advice saved up to 30 lives, and he maintains it was the right call. 'Of course it was a blow to the program,' he said. 'But in the end we got the settings right, based on the evidence.'

The Commonwealth kept tight control on the vaccines, and initially limited the role of the states. But some doses went to the wrong places, and state premiers and health ministers were publicly blasting the federal government at press conferences. At some aged-care centres and disability homes, contractors offered vaccines to residents, but left most staff unvaccinated. 'It was just a trainwreck,' Stephen Duckett, a former federal health department secretary and one of the most vocal critics of the rollout, said. 'A complete and utter shemozzle.' Duckett dubbed the rollout a 'shit-storm' at the time.

More than two years later, it is clear his view has not changed. 'We were doomed from the start because we were much, much more narrow in our investment decisions than practically every other advanced economy in the world. Other countries hedged their bets across six, seven, or eight vaccines, but we only chose four,' Duckett said.

However, Omar Khorshid has a very different view, and told us that the federal government made the right call at the time to invest in two international vaccines, Pfizer and Novavax, alongside two locally manufactured vaccines in AstraZeneca and the University of Queensland's molecular clamp. Nobody could have foreseen how effective mRNA vaccine technology (which was then brand new) was going to be, he said.

'I am not of the view that it was a vaccine "strollout". I think that's very uncharitable and easy to say in retrospect,' Khorsid said. 'Even with the benefit of hindsight, it was a pretty good and considered decision by the federal government to choose the vaccines they did. It's hard to know where we might have been if we didn't have any local manufacturing of vaccines. AstraZeneca has underpinned the bulk of our program. Yes, it's had its controversy, but it saved countless lives. People forget all of these vaccines were unproven, untested, unavailable at the time of these deals.'

The reputation of AstraZeneca was tarnished beyond repair in those early months, GP Jamal Rifi said. He still wonders, if it had not been so sullied, whether Australia might have had a chance of avoiding the punishing lockdowns that Victoria and New South Wales had to impose. 'We had AZ, which was this life-saving and highly effective vaccine, in huge supply, but the view it was inferior to Pfizer was too deeply entrenched to overcome,' he said.

The renowned Muslim leader had plans of retiring in 2020. His dream was to drive around Australia in his customised motorhome with wife, Lana. Instead, when coronavirus struck, the doctor of more than 30 years delayed his retirement. He put on his scrubs and bought two tents from Supercheap Auto, before setting up a drive-through testing clinic outside his home. 'I wanted to give back to the country that had been so good to me,' he said.

For two years, he could not see his front yard. The orange-brick–paved driveway and the circles of neatly mowed green grass in front of the doctor's home in Belmore, in south-west Sydney, were hidden beneath the two enormous tents. From behind his white-picket fence, the father-of-five and his team screened tens of thousands of Sydneysiders for the virus. 'My youngest son hated it because he had no privacy anymore,' Rifi said.

When the virulent Delta strain began to spread quickly in Sydney, Rifi felt an urgency to vaccinate his patients as fast as he could. Many resided in culturally diverse pockets of the city, and were getting infected at far higher rates than anyone else in Australia. He points out that there was no real media strategy to encourage Australians from a non-English–speaking background to get immunised, and that any health messaging distributed by governments simply was not cutting through.

Rifi said that anti-vax messaging and vaccine anxiety was

particularly widespread in Arabic-speaking and Middle Eastern communities, who were often suspicious of government authorities, due to their traumatic experiences of fleeing countries where authorities were corrupt. Research in Australia found that culturally and linguistically diverse communities reported heightened levels of anxiety, confusion, and distress, along with a greater reliance on non-official sources of information, due to the lag in public health information. Such was the level of misinformation that the Australian National Imams Council, along with the Australian Fatwa Council, felt it necessary to release an Islamic ruling deeming the Pfizer and AstraZeneca vaccines permissible under Islamic law. This followed false reports in Australia that the vaccines contained pork.

Rifi spent countless hours reassuring his patients of the benefits of the vaccine. He set up Sydney's first drive-through vaccination hub at the Canterbury-Bankstown Bulldogs football stadium, employing more than 80 staff to help. There were doctors, medical and nursing students, pharmacists, and allied health workers, led by his own son, Faisal, a registered nurse. The beauty of it was that they all spoke different languages, from Greek to Italian, Arabic, Chinese, and Vietnamese. Every day, they vaccinated 400 people from the safety of their cars. Everyone felt a sense of responsibility toward the nation in combating this virus. By the time the clinic closed its doors, Rifi and his team had vaccinated more than 30,000 people.

Rifi immunised anyone he could. When a cat was trapped between two buildings next to one of his medical clinics, he came out with a handful of vaccine vials, and personally inoculated the team of firefighters, who had come to rescue the distressed animal, on the spot. One morning, as he drove to vaccinate patients in their homes, he heard an ABC radio interview with Achieve Australia's chief executive, Jo-Anne Hewitt, expressing alarm about the more than 200 people with a disability still waiting to be vaccinated. He called into the radio station, and soon after his team vaccinated every resident.

Rifi believes that the federal government did an extraordinary job of protecting the population from a devastating death toll with measures such as early border controls, but he said Australia was let down by the shambolic, slow vaccine rollout and the absence of a culturally and linguistically diverse vaccine-education campaign. Where there should have been trust in authorities and science, there was paranoia and fear due to the tough policing measures, and confusion over the changing restrictions and health messaging, which was not cutting through to culturally diverse communities. Rifi had walked the Kokoda track with Scott Morrison in 2009, and remains a friend of the former prime minister, but he said, 'It's not tricky for me to be friends with the prime minister and say "Well done" for some things, and criticise his government at the same time. They should have done better with the vaccine messaging. I have told Scott that myself.'

He remains particularly critical of the federal government's 'arm yourself' advertising campaign, which showed a series of bare arms with Band-Aids stuck on. 'For years, we were working to counter violent extremism, and some genius in Canberra came up with the idea to say, "Arm yourself," he said. 'I thought, *How am I going to translate this in Arabic?* Arm yourself means to get a gun.'

Melbourne GP Umber Rind remembered the Victorian health department scrambling to find people to translate vaccine messages into different languages. 'There wasn't enough vaccine messaging in Arabic, or Turkish, Somali, or Vietnamese,' she said. 'They [the health department] were running around asking people to translate things, but the thing was you need proper trained interpreters to do that, so there were issues with how documents were translated.'

Rind's patients are culturally diverse, and hail from Lebanese, African, Turkish, Italian, Greek, and Asian backgrounds. She said many wanted to be vaccinated, but she did not have the supply. 'I felt there was a real inequality when it came to the number of doses allocated to certain suburbs across Melbourne.' She questioned why GPs in the affluent eastern suburbs had Pfizer available freely to give their patients, while she and her colleagues were struggling to get enough to vaccinate their most at-risk patients. The irony was that by the time vaccine supply increased in Hume in Melbourne's northern suburbs, where Rind works, the delays had led to many of her patients becoming anxious and fearful about being immunised. Some had already been misled by conspiracy theories, a situation worsened by supporters of Australian businessman Clive Palmer distributing pamphlets in letterboxes in Hume, questioning the efficacy of the vaccine. 'For some of them, it was very hard to convince them; but for others, the outbreak quickly changed their mind when they saw people they knew getting really sick, or even dying,' she recalled.

In Hume, coronavirus was spreading like wildfire in the winter of 2021—something that could not simply be explained by recalcitrant rule-breakers breaching lockdown restrictions. At the peak of the wave, Victoria's Covid-19 commander, Jeroen Weimar, revealed that more than half of the transmission in the local government area of Hume was occurring within the home, and the remaining infections were the result of social interactions between households, such as someone visiting their relatives or elderly parents.

Hume, with its densely populated suburbs, and home to more than 240,000 people, was reporting more than one-third of all infections in Melbourne. Complicating the matter was the fact that 54 per cent of Hume's workforce were essential workers who needed to travel for their jobs. Many were young and mobile, and yet they had not been prioritised for vaccinations. There were high numbers of multi-generational families, too, living together and often crammed under the one roof; one in ten homes during the pandemic had more than eight occupants. Yet, despite this, Hume had a shortage of doctors, and its access to vaccines was amongst the lowest in Victoria.

As soon as the federal government declared in February 2021 that general practice clinics would be the cornerstone of Australia's vaccination scheme, the rollout was doomed to be inequitable. When it became clear that vaccines were not being rolled out fast enough, the Victorian government took the reins, establishing a drive-through vaccination clinic at the old Ford factory in Broadmeadows, and a new walk-in and pop-up clinic in Hume, escalating the availability of vaccinations by tens of thousands. As the risk of getting infected with the Delta variant rose, thousands of young Victorians under the age of 40, who were not yet approved for Pfizer doses, weighed up their own individual risk, and began rolling up their sleeves for AstraZeneca. Intervals between doses were shortened by ATAGI to hasten the number of Australians fully vaccinated with two doses. Across Melbourne, vaccine pop-up clinics began emerging in trusted venues such as churches, schools, and mosques.

During the Delta outbreak, the Austin Hospital's entire intensive-care ward was occupied by patients with a Middle Eastern or Arabic background who were unvaccinated and lived in Melbourne's northern suburbs. The Austin's director of intensive care, Stephen Warrillow, said it was a situation that doctors in Australia had never seen before. 'We had to do this terribly delicate dance of putting community messaging out to people about being vaccinated, who might not, for no fault of their own, engage with mainstream media without stigmatising them,' Warrillow said. 'This was a disease of everybody. We had to do it in a way without implying that somehow these people are at fault.'

People that general practitioner Umber Rind knew personally had been hospitalised, compelling her to take to social media, and to share a series of harrowing posts, begging people to get vaccinated. 'I felt anger, disappointment, then I just felt really sad,' Rind said. 'It was all so predictable. It still makes me so upset that our area in the north was not targeted for vaccines earlier.'

Warrillow recalled Dr Ahmad Aly, a gastrointestinal surgeon at Melbourne's Austin Hospital, calling him out of the blue and asking to visit the ICU. Egyptian-born Aly, who is the brother of academic and co-host of *The Project* Waleed Aly, asked if he could film a video inside the ICU to show his community the reality of the deadly disease. Warrillow said that Ahmad Aly was shocked and distressed by what he saw. Later, he made an impassioned plea. 'They're young, they're not vaccinated, they are all from our community,' he said in the video. 'Please, please, if you are a leader here, if you have influence … you have to tell your people, our community, to get vaccinated.' The video went viral being viewed hundreds of thousands of times, and triggering a much-needed surge in vaccinations in the north.

In New South Wales, a similar troubling trend was unfolding in hospitals. When Khaled Elmasri, a mover and shaker in New South Wales' Muslim community, was hospitalised with the virus, Rifi asked Khaled to send him a message that he could share publicly. 'Two days later, he sent me this unscripted video—it was coming from the heart,' he said. Speaking in Arabic from his hospital bed, wheezing and gasping for breath, Khaled said, 'I have learnt my lesson the hard way, and now I'm going to get the vaccine.' In the following days, Rifi said, vaccine bookings across Sydney soared.

The success of Australia's Covid-19 vaccine rollout heavily relied on the goodwill of general practitioners such as Rifi and Rind, and on community leaders such as Ahmad Malas. Research would later find that participation in the Covid-19 vaccine rollout resulted in increased stress and immense financial instability for general practitioners. For months, Rifi's phone did not stop ringing. Hundreds of calls poured in from people asking him to vaccinate them at their home. Unless he knew the family well, Rifi never went alone, anxious that there might be someone waiting to ambush him. His fears were warranted. There were many occasions when he ended up in tense confrontations with adult children of elderly patients who did not want their parents vaccinated. When he posted a photograph of himself being vaccinated on social media, he was trolled online viciously, and received a barrage of death threats. 'I was called all sorts of names,' Rifi said. 'We had vaccination signs out the front of the clinics smashed. Staff were threatened, and the police were called several times.'

But he has never been one to shy away from his beliefs. After the Cronulla riots in 2005, when he spoke out to promote peace, he recalled being 'able to taste the hate that was engulfing and motivating these people'. In 2015, he received death threats after publicly denouncing Islamic State. When the terrorist organisation posted a photo of the young son of Australian ISIS fighter Khaled Sharrouf holding a severed head, Rifi described Sharrouf as 'a despicable person'. He told us that, 'There is a link between my work that I have done against extremism in the past and the work against coronavirus. They both are killers, and they both are nasty. One is a virus; the other one is an ideology. But both of them are very damaging to the common decent human being.'

For many months in 2021, Rifi collapsed from exhaustion each night. He lay in bed reading motorhome brochures, dreaming of his escape. But the toll of the pandemic crept up suddenly. By December, Rifi was struggling to get out of bed. 'I felt that I had a really dark cloud over my head,' he said. 'I felt unlike myself. At first, I started hating seeing and talking to people. Then I started to hate myself.'

Rifi still finds it difficult to untangle his feelings from back then. He was bone-achingly tired, beyond burnt out, but there was such a deep sadness, too. He found himself crying inconsolably for days on end. The doctor stopped working, and moved to his holiday home on the central coast in New South Wales. 'It cleansed my soul. But it was a terrible time,' Rifi said. 'Some days, the tears just wouldn't stop. I realised I was grieving. I had many of my patients die during the pandemic. Family members died, friends I had known my whole life, and I couldn't grieve for them because I was in the midst of things. There was so much pain in my heart. I grieved all the unnecessary deaths of my patients who would not get vaccinated and got infected and died. The ones who didn't call the ambulance because they were afraid to go to hospital. I could not pay my respects to them. There were so many close to my heart.'

For almost five months, while Rifi lived by the sea, he kept his phone switched off. His days were filled with tending to the garden, planting native Australian trees, and bird watching. He found solace in the warmth of the sun and the smell of the air just before it rained. The dark cloud finally lifted when he reunited with his brother in

Turkey in 2022 after more than three years apart. 'There were no more tears for what seemed the longest time,' he said. 'There was just happiness in my heart.'

Back in Queensland, AstraZeneca was hit by another grenade when the state's chief health officer, Jeannette Young, attracted a storm of criticism after publicly challenging a decision announced by Morrison to open the door for Australians under the age of 40 to get the AstraZeneca vaccine. Morrison had intended to speed up the vaccine rollout and to allow young people, who were not yet eligible for a vaccine, the chance to be inoculated with AstraZeneca once they had weighed up their individual risk with their doctor. On 1 July 2021, during another late-night press conference inside The Lodge, where he was quarantining after a work trip, Morrison announced an indemnity scheme for doctors who might want to give the AstraZeneca vaccine to younger Australians. But the next day, Young poured cold water all over it.

'I do not want under-40s to get AstraZeneca,' an aghast Young, who seemed to be at the end her tether, said during a televised press conference. 'I don't want an 18-year-old in Queensland dying from a clotting illness who, if they got Covid, probably wouldn't die.' Young said she did not understand why Mr Morrison had departed from the advice of ATAGI. 'We are not in a position that I need to ask young, fit, healthy people to put their health on the line by getting a vaccine that could, potentially, significantly harm them.'

Fellow experts, as well as political figures and commentators, turned on her. But Young, though privately deeply upset by the controversy, stuck to her position. She had been inoculated with AstraZeneca, but was accused of fuelling the anti-vax movement. Posters put up around Melbourne featured an image of Young and the quote: 'I don't want an 18-year-old in Queensland dying from a clotting illness who, if they got Covid, probably wouldn't die.' Paul Griffin, an infectious disease expert in Brisbane, who has been the principal investigator for seven Covid-19 vaccine clinical trials, including for AstraZeneca, said that Young's comments, coming from a highly respected figure in Queensland, did irreparable damage.

'It did two things: it made people under-appreciate the risk of Covid, and it increased their perception of risk around vaccines,' Griffin said. 'It also had an impact on the uptake of other vaccines. Queensland remains the lowest in terms of vaccines per head of population in the country, and we really struggled to get our booster uptake up.'

Behind the scenes, in early 2021, Professor James McCaw said some politicians were making the case to reopen Australia's international borders once 50 per cent of the adult population had been inoculated. 'It was very close ... they walked up to the edge and had a look over it,' said McCaw, then a member of the Australian Health Protection Principal Committee. Such a move would have squandered almost every gain made in suppressing the virus through enforcing some of the world's strictest border rules and punishing lockdowns, McCaw said. That high-stakes period was one of the few times during the pandemic that the level-headed McCaw felt 'really stressed.'

'There was a view in government, and you heard the rhetoric in the media too at that time, that if we have vaccinated half the population, we can open the borders because we have halved the risk.' In the end, McCaw said the federal government took the advice of advisers such as himself who presented the scientific evidence of what could unfold if Australia were to abandon its Covid-zero strategy with just half of the eligible population vaccinated. 'They pushed back. Then they listened, and they changed their view. We had a good outcome,' he said. 'But it felt like it was really close. Like, we just kept thinking we've got to make sure we get this across.'

By 20 October 2021, 70 per cent of Australians over the age of 16 had received two vaccine doses, hitting the target of inoculations set by the federal government. It was a moment of triumph, signalling the beginning of a slow easing of restrictions under the national plan for reopening. But there was a great variation in the states' vaccination rates, causing a more staggered release. Victoria hit 70 per cent just in time for the October milestone, while New South Wales and Canberra had just surpassed 80 per cent double-dose rates. Unsurprisingly, states less affected by coronavirus lockdowns, including Western Australia, Queensland, and the Northern Territory, did not reach their 70 per cent milestones until mid-November. This meant that some states, like Western Australia, would not open their borders to the rest of the country for many more months, causing tension between its government and the Commonwealth.

The director of the Doherty Institute, Professor Sharon Lewin, said the milestone heralded a move away from a Covid-zero approach for many states, including Victoria. A consortium of modellers, led by the institute, were the architects of a report underpinning the Morrison government's reopening of Australia after two years as a 'fortress nation.' It was a mammoth job, and the stakes were immense. Lewin remembers the anxiety around the release of the documents. As the spokeswoman for the institute, she did her best to shield her staff from the scrutiny.

'Questions were being raised about where Doherty was positioned,' Lewin said. 'It was an incredibly stressful time. We're a scientific organisation. We are not public policy or the government. We would never compromise what we do. We provide information on data and science to governments to make decisions. That line was getting very blurred in September [2021].'

It was the scientific modellers who had deemed that all states could begin relaxing lockdowns and restrictions when 70 per cent of the population was vaccinated. The first phase of the plan included the abolition of caps on vaccinated Australians returning from overseas, and the lifting of all restrictions on outbound travel for vaccinated Australians. Further freedoms were to be granted at 80 per cent and beyond. But as Australia inched close to the 70 per cent milestone, hundreds of coronavirus cases were still being reported each week, raising concerns that the long-awaited reopening might be delayed. There were days of debate between state premiers, prime minister Scott Morrison, and epidemiologists over whether the targets were still appropriate, given the magnitude of New South Wales' outbreak.

This prompted Lewin to declare that whether Australia opened at '30 cases or 800 cases,' the nation could still open up safely with 70 to 80 per cent vaccination rates. 'It might seem that these 'test, trace, isolate, and quarantine' measures aren't currently working in New South Wales or Victoria. But they are,' Lewin told the ABC in August 2021 as debate raged. 'They are stopping transmissions, and reducing the effective reproduction rate from 5 to closer to 1.3 in New South Wales.'

Morrison remembers hours-long national cabinet meetings debating the national plan with the state leaders in 2021. He would tune into the video calls from his study in The Lodge, where he was often tending a log fire to ward off the bitter Canberra cold. 'The premiers were very amused by the fact I had to get up every few minutes to put the fire on and tend to it,' Morrison said. 'I think Mark McGowan said, "It looks like you're in Batman's lair."'

But for all the chaos, heartache, and confusion of Australia's national vaccine rollout, Professor Robert Booy, an epidemiologist and infectious disease expert from the University of Sydney, said that Australia eventually became a global leader in immunisation. 'In the end, we got there,' Booy said. 'We have to remember the rate of death we got per head per population in the first two years of the pandemic in Australia was ten times lower than many countries like the US and the UK. Eventually we had among the highest vaccination rates in the world.'

CHAPTER SIXTEEN

An ocean of conspiracies

Canberra's Covid-zero days were numbered. It had been more than a year since Australia's smallest jurisdiction had reported a local infection: 398 days, to be precise. But with cases of the infectious Delta strain climbing steadily in neighbouring New South Wales, coronavirus was closing in on the Australian capital, the home of Australia's federal parliament. 'We kind of sit as an island in the middle of New South Wales,' explained the Australian Capital Territory's chief health officer, Dr Kerryn Coleman. 'I think we all knew it was inevitable it would appear.'

The positive case that broke the Covid-zero streak on 12 August 2021 was a Commonwealth Games wrestler and local bouncer. Rumours circulated that the man in his 20s had made an illegal trip to Sydney, where he had picked up the disease, but Coleman said, 'This bloke did everything we asked him, despite a vicious response [from the public].' ACT chief minister Andrew Barr said it wasn't even certain that the bouncer was patient zero in the outbreak, which quickly began growing, and caused the territory and its population of about 430,000 people to join New South Wales and Victoria in lockdowns.

It was during one of the daily Covid press conferences that followed when the internet sensation 'Ken Behrens' was born. The event was being transcribed by a Sydney captioning company when a mistake slipped through. The chief minister of the ACT was saying he wanted 'to thank Canberrans for doing the right thing'. But the subtitles that went to air read, 'I want to thank *Ken Behrens* for doing the right thing'. The error delighted social media, and instantly spawned a new nickname for residents of Australia's small capital. ACT Policing tweeted: 'I am staying at home. I am only leaving home for essential reasons. I am wearing a mask whenever I go outside. I am Ken Behrens.' The operator responsible for the mistake told local radio that when he saw a post about the error, he initially thought someone else had made the typo. 'I was sort of sitting there, thinking, *Yeah I'll get the juicy goss*', he joked. 'As soon as I saw the screenshot, I just had that heart-sinking moment.'

Canberra also made headlines for its impressive vaccination rates. In November 2021, official government data showed that 100 per cent of the ACT's adult population had received their first Covid-19 inoculation. But then the vaccination rate kept climbing higher. In some age categories, Barr said the data showed that up to 115 per cent of the population had 'been vaccinated'. The simple explanation for the impossibly high figure was that the population estimate for the ACT had not accounted for growth, possibly by around 20,000 extra people, or about 5 per cent. However, Barr believes that, even with the anomalies, the ACT was the most vaccinated jurisdiction in the nation, an achievement he credits partly to the small size of the city-state, as 'it wasn't too far to go to get a vaccine', and to the high education levels of the city, which is home to tens of thousands of government workers.

There was a point in August 2021 when roughly 15 million Australians were back in lockdown as several states fought incursions of the Delta strain. Melbourne went into its sixth shutdown on 5 August. It was only meant to last seven days. Instead, it stretched to 77. Earlier that year, Victoria authorities had had success in containing a string of outbreaks with snap lockdowns and rigorous testing, contact tracing, and quarantine. In fact, the weary city had already batted back two Delta outbreaks, including one sparked by contagious furniture removalists from Sydney who had lugged a mattress and other furniture into an apartment building in Melbourne in July. Many assumed that this new and final Delta outbreak, which surfaced with a teacher and a warehouse worker, was simply part of the preceding cluster of cases. But genomics investigations showed that it was very likely to be a new incursion. By the time Victoria reopened again on 21 October 2021, Melbourne had been shut down for 262 days, longer than any other major city in the world.

Associate Professor James Trauer, the head of the epidemiological modelling unit at Monash University, said he was frustrated by the lighter approach of New South Wales to the notoriously dangerous Delta variant. 'I felt like New South Wales were just messing around, because there were so many reasons to go hard at that point,' he said. 'They refused to adopt the strategy of the rest of the country, which in hindsight might have avoided a second prolonged lockdown in Melbourne.'

Trauer, who lived in Melbourne, said almost every Australian state had, in effect, an elimination approach by the latter part of 2020. They would bring in lockdowns early, with the aim of shutting down outbreaks quickly. New South Wales was the outlier, using lockdowns later and more reluctantly, while still aiming to have no Covid spreading in the community. New South Wales premier Gladys Berejiklian explained in January 2021 that the goal was still to have no Covid spreading in the community, 'but we do it in a way which doesn't overburden our citizens every single day'.

Victoria's health minister, Martin Foley, said he knew the initial partial lockdown of Sydney was not going to work, and he shared this view with his close confidant, New South Wales' health minister, Brad Hazzard. But Foley also said he understood why the New South Wales government took a softer approach than Victoria did. 'Did I understand why they did? Absolutely. Because they'd seen the way we've been pilloried. And they saw the pressure that we've been under the previous year.'

On 6 August, as cases of the Delta strain surged past 4,500 in New South Wales, premier Gladys Berejiklian acknowledged that eradicating the outbreak was slipping out of reach. Eliminating it had become an aspiration, she said, rather than a goal. 'We know, given where the numbers are and the experience of Delta overseas, that we now have to live with Delta in one way or another—and that's pretty obvious.'

The Victorian government held onto the goal of eradication a little longer, clamping down on 'rule bending' by lockdown-fatigued residents by banning them from removing their masks in public, after reports emerged of people sipping takeaway cocktails on the street. Playgrounds were again cordoned off. Victorian premier Daniel Andrews berated people for using the exercise allowances as 'an opportunity for seven families to catch up in the park'. But despite everything Victorian authorities threw at the outbreak, it kept growing. 'It's now clear to us that we are not going to drive these numbers down—they are instead going to increase,' Andrews said on 1 September 2021.

The declaration that Victoria would no longer pursue Covid zero was an emotional moment for many Victorians who had sacrificed so much, again and again, to eradicate outbreaks. But by this time, the state had already achieved something that at times looked impossible: buying Victoria and the rest of the country valuable time for vaccination. It saved many lives. Underlining this, the death rate in New South Wales' second wave was about ten times lower than in Victoria's 2020 outbreak. The virus wasn't any less deadly; instead, authorities had had time to largely ring-fence nursing homes and the country's older population with vaccinations.

Whenever Victoria's chief health officer, Brett Sutton, has contemplated the alternative—a less restrictive approach that did not rely heavily on lockdowns, and allowed for transmission to circulate—he always comes back to what it could have meant, not only for Victoria but the rest of the country. In the scenario that Victoria had failed to defeat the second wave of disease, 'it would have meant thousands upon thousands of deaths in Victoria'. Knowing what he knows now, about the added threat of long-term complications for those who are unvaccinated, as well as the heightened risk of other diseases—respiratory, cardiac, and neurological complications following the virus—has only strengthened Sutton's view it was the right decision.

'Clearly, it was impossibly hard, and clearly it harmed populations, and it harmed individuals economically, psychologically, [and] physically because of the constraints on our movements, and the constraints on our freedoms and the limit on our interactions,' Sutton said. But without the restrictions imposed on Victorians, Sutton said that Covid would have breached the boundaries of other Australia states, irrespective of border closures. 'I think there would have been another 30,0000 or 40,000 deaths in Australia, because they couldn't have contained it to Victoria.'

As the Covid-zero dream was declared dead in Australia's most populous states, the challenge moved to suppressing the outbreaks so their hospitals would not run out of beds. In line with national policy, the New South Wales, Victorian, and Australian Capital Territory governments resolved to begin lifting their lockdowns once about 70 per cent of adults had been double vaccinated. In an effort to speed up the reopening, large parts of the population, including teachers, police, and construction workers, were required to get two vaccine doses to be allowed to work. For a while, people even had to show their vaccination record to go out for dinner, or to get a haircut. While the hardline approach helped push up the nation's vaccination rate to extremely high levels, it also bred deep resentment among people who felt coerced or locked out.

Some of the fury and resentment that had been simmering just below the surface erupted on 21 September 2021 during Melbourne's sixth lockdown. The city's Westgate Bridge was stormed by hundreds of construction workers and other men dressed in high-vis work gear. Some set off flares, threw objects at cars, or jumped onto the trays of passing trucks as television helicopters hummed above them. At one point, the protestors broke out into a rendition of the song 'Horses', made famous by Australian musician Daryl Braithwaite.

The protests were, at least partly, an emotional reaction to the Victorian government's decision to mandate vaccines on construction sites, and to temporarily shut down the building sector over Covid rule-breaking. But the chaos was also symbolic of the parlous state of the morale of locked-down Melbourne, and the intense strangeness of the time. In a place that mostly prided itself on peaceful resistance, a mob was seen at the outskirts of the CBD chasing down and bashing police cars, smashing a back window, and trying to prise off a rear-view mirror. Sirens wailed.

The next morning, something else happened that was monumental enough to briefly knock the news of the protests off the top of the television bulletins. The city was struck by a magnitude-5.9 earthquake. It was the largest onshore tremor ever recorded in Victoria, strong enough to visibly rattle people's homes. No one was hurt, but dozens of buildings were damaged, and it brought down half a wall in an inner-city shipping strip. 'What's next?' people joked wryly. 'A plague of locusts?'

There were no locusts; instead, several hundred protestors descended on the Shrine of Remembrance, a venerated monument in Melbourne honouring the service and sacrifice of Australians in war and peacekeeping. It is usually a site of quiet reflection and respect for the fallen, set within gardens on the southern edge of the city. In an hours-long standoff, demonstrators stood and sat on the steps of the shrine, chanting, and waving flags and banners.

Burned into television journalist Paul Dowsley's memory of this day was the heavy police presence that felt odd in Melbourne: the heavy armoured vehicles, police horses clattering down the street, and loud bangs echoing off the apartment buildings on St Kilda Road. 'Can you hear the shots?' Dowsley asked the anchor back in the Seven News studio, as he reported from the protest site and a huge contingent of police, wearing helmets and bullet-proof vests, moved on the group, firing rubber bullets. Smoke hung in the air. Flares were let off by protestors. Later, urine was found on the walls of the monument, and rubbish was scattered on the lawns around it.

The day before, Dowsley had been attacked by four people while covering the riotous protests. The reporter was grabbed around the neck and pinned against a steel rubbish bin by several men while he was following the crowd surging through Melbourne's CBD. He was spat on. Urine was splashed in his face, and on the cameraman, too. 'I reckon for half an hour, we were spitting it out,' Dowsley said. 'I can tell you, it sticks around.' Soon after, he was struck while live on air with an energy drink can that had been hurled from a distance away, leaving him with a small cut on the back of his head. 'On reflection, you kind of go, *Geez, that was unprecedented*,' Dowsley said. 'It's a word that gets thrown around probably too much, but certainly in my career it was unprecedented.'

Protests against Covid lockdowns and vaccines persisted in one form or another for several years, in many capital cities — often held on a Saturday, and sometimes disturbed by violent clashes with police. For a time, one of the people at the front of the throng was Ash Jackson. Before the pandemic, the musician, who was in her late 40s, had been earning a living playing in pub bands around Melbourne, and teaching guitar. But during the city's second lockdown in 2020, she found herself unable to work and living alone in her St Kilda apartment. Her window to the world was the internet, and she spent almost all her waking hours lost in some of its darker corners. She started believing outlandish QAnon conspiracies peddled on YouTube videos: that children were being sold and trafficked using coded language on the website of a furniture company.

'I was even a fan of [US President] Donald Trump, which is ridiculous,' she said. 'I'm transgender, and he's not very favourable to us. But in that community, you either believe everything, or you get shunned out.' Increasingly, Victoria Police became the focus of much of Jackson's anger and distorted beliefs. At protests, she would swear and scream at them, telling them 'How good was Walsh Street?'—a reference to the shooting murder of two young police officers in Melbourne in 1988. 'The feeling at that point … was that we needed to form an underground resistance against the police and government, which is crazy, I know,' she said.

Jackson wrote an instruction book that described counter tactics that could be used against police, which she later described as 'almost like a terrorism' document. However, it was her interaction with law enforcement that eventually opened the door to Jackson's escape from the movement. In the back of her mind there had always been a bit of doubt, and when a series of individual officers treated Jackson with compassion, the doubt spilled over. During the last freedom protest she attended in May 2021, Jackson had been with a small group of protestors near Victoria Market marching towards police when she realised her friends had fled, leaving her alone. But the police let her off with a move-on order, because they said she had been cooperative. The following week, when Jackson was arrested at home and taken in for questioning about her role in the anti-lockdown protest movement, they empathised with her concerns, saying, 'We've got families, too. Our job isn't to make policy.'

Detectives would continue dropping in at her house for a while, showing interest in a book she was writing. 'They said, "Ash, if you ever have a feeling like you want to go back, or you need help with something, just pop into the station. If we've got some time, we'll sit down and have a coffee."' Jackson had fallen out with many of her friends and her family, but at Christmas that year she got a call from her brother, saying he wanted her to come for lunch. 'The biggest moving part for me was seeing my nieces,' she said. 'Just seeing them again was amazing.'

The identity of the freedom protestors was often subject to debate. Were these people real tradies, or opportunistic neo-Nazis in steel-capped boots? Were they devastated mums and dads who had lost their businesses, or crazed conspiracy theorists? *Sunday Age* reporter Rachael Dexter closely followed what became known as the freedom movement in Melbourne. What she experienced as she covered the illegal marches was a miscellany of all of these groups, very loosely united in protest. There were tradies from the suburbs, vaccine-sceptical 'natural medicine' mothers, retirees, high-school students, families with toddlers, people in suits, and small-business owners. People yelled that the vaccines contained microchips, controlled by 5G technology. Others claimed that Victorian premier Daniel Andrews and his family were living in tunnels underneath Crown Casino.

Dexter said there was no coherent list of grievances that pulled all these people together, not even opposition to vaccination. Illustrating this broad church of frustration with authorities, Dexter remembers seeing a people-mover car, like something a mum would drive on the school run, parked in the CBD during one of the marches. Written in liquid chalk on the rear windscreen were the words: 'No more lockdowns. My kids need school. I need to work.' Perhaps if there was any unifying force, reflected Dexter, it was a collective 'push back'.

When the last lockdown was lifted in Victoria in 2021, there was a noticeable drop in protest attendees as people headed back to their jobs. Many groups and individuals tried to capitalise politically and financially on the movement, with various success. But no single leader emerged, and QAnon-style conspiracies about child sacrifice, while present, weren't widely embraced. 'You could hear it in the crowd sometimes. A speaker would get up and start dropping QAnon messages, and you could see some people in the crowd thinking, *What the hell is going on here?*, or they were trying to conduct a mass prayer, and there were gym bros booing in the back,' Dexter said. 'I think the difference in Australia compared to America is we didn't have that Trump-type figurehead. There's still a lot of healthy scepticism.'

However, the conspiracy movement did see escalating death threats against Australian politicians. Anti-terrorist police quietly charged a number of people associated with the Melbourne protests, including a man who encouraged demonstrators to bring guns and to use them to execute the Victorian premier, Daniel Andrews.

Martin Foley, the Victorian health minister, said that he and his colleagues had security patrolling their homes around the clock. The seasoned MP was accustomed to abuse on social media, but it was the 'scary' looking people approaching him and his children on the streets that left him fearing for his life and his family's safety. 'When your kids come home and tell you … and they're pretty resilient—kids of MPs have to be—but when they tell you that people come up to them on the street and have a go, that's tough,' he said.

A package 'with wires and stuff sticking out of it' was sent to his Port Melbourne electorate office in the spring of 2021. The surrounding streets were cordoned off, and a bomb squad robot was wheeled in to dismantle the package, soon determined to be a hoax. Foley said threats intensified to such a point that he asked not to be fully briefed on them, preferring not to know the full extent of the danger he was facing.

Conspiracy theorists would also cast doubt on the cause of an accident when Daniel Andrews slipped and injured his back on the wooden steps of a Sorrento holiday home on 9 March 2021. The injuries led to Andrews being hooked up to a breathing machine for two days in the Alfred Hospital in Melbourne, battling respiratory failure due to several broken ribs and damaged vertebrae. 'It was awful,' recalled his wife, Catherine, who said she thought her husband was going to die when she found him groaning in pain, turning blue.

A bedridden Andrews was forced to take 111 days off work, abruptly ending his near-constant presence in the lives of Victorians through his daily coronavirus press conferences. James Merlino, who was the deputy premier and education minister, stepped in until Andrews returned on 28 June.

Speculation about the premier's fall was rife for months, spread via messages on the encrypted social media app Telegram and an article on a Queensland blog with the title 'Who bashed Dan Andrews?'. The blog claimed the injuries suffered by the premier

were 'consistent with having been kicked while prone on the ground'.
The same website has promoted stories that the pandemic was fabri-
cated by the World Health Organisation and that Covid-19 vaccines
caused a spate of car accidents and countless other deaths. Although
the Andrews accident theories proved only to be mischief-making,
Victorian Liberal politician Louise Staley would further fan the
flames of speculation when she issued a press release demanding
the premier answer a list of 12 questions about the accident to prove
there was no 'cover up'.

Around the same time, Professor Catherine Bennett, an epidemiologist who became well known in Australia for her prolific media
appearances discussing Covid, was also having her emails screened
by her employer, Deakin University, for security purposes. On at least
one occasion, the university was concerned enough to contact police.
However, she also often engaged with those who, having taken
umbrage with something she had said, rang her, and were shocked
to discover that Bennett answered her own work phone. 'They were
probably going to leave a disparaging remark about vaccines, but
when I talked to them and I answered their questions, they'd say,
"That's really cool,"' she recalled. 'I learnt so much about what people
were worried about.'

As the early pandemic-conspiracy theories began doing the
rounds, Bennett decided to make herself available to a spectrum
of media outlets, ranging from the BBC to Australia's conservative
news channel, Sky News. During lockdowns, Bennett said, she
worked 100 hours a week, researching and doing up to 25 media
interviews daily. It was not unusual for her day to start well before
dawn, when she would begin prepping at 5.00 am for breakfast-tele-
vision appearances. Often, the networks would send a camera to her
house, and she would stand on her front lawn in Melbourne's north,
in freezing conditions or while being bitten by mosquitoes. Many
other interviews were done as Bennett sat in her dining room in the
middle of her house, in front of a cabinet topped with an old radio
from her childhood.

Almost immediately after she began appearing on television, the epidemiologist was recognised when out and about in her neighbourhood. For a little while, people didn't say anything, although she clocked the recognition in their faces. Then, one day, while at the post office, the manager loudly declared, 'You're looking good on television.' All the other customers looked up and stared at her.

The fame stuck around even when Covid-19 slipped off the newspapers' front pages. It was near impossible for the scientist to go anywhere in Australia without being recognised—a task made harder by her distinctive appearance. Bennett's dark, curly hair is topped with a natural streak of grey, and she has a voice made for radio.

One day, she was leaving a small café when she noticed a man lingering at the doorway of the restaurant. 'I was just wondering if I could buy you a drink,' he said. *How weird*, Bennett thought. The epidemiologist was not feeling herself, and hadn't been expecting to be asked out. She spent the first few years of the pandemic unable to keep up her usual exercise routine as she battled lingering fatigue and shortness of breath from a nasty respiratory infection caught on an international flight in late 2019.

Slightly flustered, Bennett replied that her partner was waiting outside. The man told her that he 'just wanted to figure out a way to say thank you', and Bennett realised that his offer was to do with her Covid media appearances. It was lovely to know that people valued and felt reassured by her commentary and advice during the pandemic, she said, but it was hard if you could never escape it. 'I tie my hair up, I wear it out, you try different things, but you don't realise how distinctive you are until you try to go incognito.'

As Covid conspiracies and vaccine hesitancy spilled into the street protests in the spring of 2021, those with anti-vaccine beliefs started being admitted to hospitals, sometimes with tragic results. In 2021, Royal Melbourne Hospital nursing manager Michelle Spence's eyes filled with tears and her voice wavered as she addressed journalists during one of Victoria's daily Covid press conferences. 'We have had people die in our intensive-care units by themselves, and we held their hands while their families had to be at home,' Spence said. Increasingly, the senior nurse said, she was caring for younger people with Covid who were begging to be vaccinated moments before they were intubated and hooked up to life support, unsure they would survive the disease.

The patients who filled Australia's isolation wards in the first 18 months of the pandemic were disproportionately returned travellers, essential workers, or old, frail people from aged-care homes. But when the Delta variant hit, many of the patients were middle-aged and otherwise healthy. By September 2021, the median age of Covid patients at the Royal Melbourne Hospital was 46. The year before, it had been over 60. Rows of unconscious people filled ICU wards. They were ventilated and laid on their stomachs in what is known as the prone position, a lifesaving treatment that helps to increase the amount of oxygen getting into the lungs when a person is in acute respiratory distress. Tiny resuscitation tables were brought into the ICUs for newborn babies, following a rise in pregnant, unvaccinated women who were infected and admitted to hospital. Often, there were multiple family members of the same family receiving care at the same time.

'There were couples in their 30s or 40s in the ICU with kids at primary and early secondary school. These kids were at risk of both their parents dying,' said Associate Professor Stephen Warrillow, the director of intensive care at the Austin Hospital, in Melbourne's northern suburbs. The physician endured the most challenging days of his 20-year career during the Delta wave, working 18-hour days. The majority of the families were gracious and kind, but some relatives of the unvaccinated patients who did not believe the virus was real made threats against him and his staff. They told him, 'If Covid is on the death certificate, there will be consequences.' Warrillow put this aggression down to families not being allowed into the

ICU because of strict infection-control protocols, which meant that communication was only via FaceTime and phone calls.

He described conversations he had with a woman whose husband was gravely ill. 'She was a very loving spouse and intelligent person, but she had been very caught up in this whole conspiracy ocean,' he said. 'She kept sending us articles and all sorts of things suggesting that a massive dose of Vitamin C works, and we were gently trying to convey to her, without brutalising her, that her husband was dying.' The woman finally asked if there was anything she could have done to prevent it. 'I said the only treatment we have that we know that can prevent this is the vaccine,' he said. 'You could almost hear the penny drop and that moment of sudden realisation. She began begging for him to be vaccinated, but it was too late.'

Warrillow said the realisation that the virus was real was often compounded by the shame of not having encouraged the person to be vaccinated, or even a feeling of immense guilt for being the person who had unwittingly exposed somebody they loved to the virus. 'To accept the truth is to accept that this didn't need to happen, and what a horrific, terrible realisation that would be,' he said. 'I cannot imagine how that would feel to have the person that you cared about most in the world dying from something that was within your power to have prevented. There would not be much that was more confronting than that.'

Instead of asking for approved treatments, families started requesting ivermectin, a veterinary drug used to treat human afflictions such as parasitic worms, head lice, and rosacea. Others demanded the anti-malaria drug hydroxychloroquine, which became a remedy of choice for Covid deniers when it was embraced by US president Donald Trump, despite it being ineffective in treating Covid and warnings that it could cause heart problems. Some believed that their loved one was being used as a part of a global experiment, or was being intentionally poisoned by healthcare workers.

Associate Professor Craig French, the director of intensive care at Western Health, which oversees Footscray and Sunshine hospital in Melbourne, said the level of verbal assault his staff were exposed to was something he had never experienced before: 'The misinformation, the belief it wasn't real, the absolute distress experienced by them when their relatives were critically unwell, made it very, very difficult to have a conversation with them about how we could help them, because what they were requesting was not consistent with the medical advice.'

French said he had to change his style of speaking when he called the families of patients who needed to be ventilated, if they were to have any chance of survival. He said his tone became less inclusive and more autocratic. 'I remember saying to a certain family [of a dying, unvaccinated patient], "I am the doctor, I am the expert. This is the recommended treatment, this is what we are going to do, or they will die" sort of thing,' French said. 'We were trying to save people's lives. But if you showed any sign of hesitation, from their perspective it would be perceived as a weakness, and they would become more aggressive.'

French holds the view that vaccination is an individual choice, and irrespective of whether a person was immunised or not, they always received the same level of care in his ICU ward. 'We didn't judge, we just got on with the job,' he said. 'But it was so hard. It was a tragedy to watch people die who just didn't need to. I looked after many people who weren't vaccinated and who died, and the reality is if they'd been vaccinated, way fewer of them would have died.'

Many patients had hypoxemia as coronavirus starved their lungs of oxygen and triggered multi-organ failure. X-rays of patients showed lungs that looked white as a bone, indicating that they almost had no air-filled spaces to breathe through. Western Health treated the most Victorians infected with Covid-19 in 2020. However, the more virulent Delta variant meant that staff treated more coronavirus patients in three months of 2021 than during the entirety of 2020.

Western Health's critical care nurse Louise Watson, who worked in the ICU ward at Sunshine Hospital when Delta hit, had cared for countless patients with pneumonia over the years, yet nothing prepared her for what she saw. It was the primal and desperate hunger for air that stayed in her mind. 'The people are just so severely depleted of oxygen, they are literally gasping for air,' Watson said during the height of the Delta outbreak in 2021. 'They have such panic in their eyes. What we were having to tolerate in terms of oxygen levels that patients experienced is something I have never seen before.'

Years later, Watson would still think back to coronavirus patients from this time and wonder if they had survived, such as the unvaccinated new mother who had recently given birth. The woman was sedated, hooked up to a ventilator, and about to be transferred to an ECMO machine (where an artificial lung is used to breathe for patients) when Watson arranged to video-call the young mother's family using an iPad.

'The husband was holding this newborn baby in his arms,' Watson recalled. 'The little children were trying to reach through the screen to touch her. As a mother myself, it broke my heart. It was just terrible. She was very close to dying.'

Another day, she performed CPR for half an hour on a man who had come into the hospital for a hip replacement, only to catch Covid. She watched him turning grey as he went into respiratory distress. By the time he died, some of his family had not seen him for 40 days, because hospitals were limiting visitors.

'Often, we didn't know what treatment was going to work, so we were just flogging everything we could to try and save people,' the mother-of-two said. 'It is hard to think about how many people's lives were changed forever during that time. There were so many families where multiple members died within days of each other.'

In 2021, French became increasingly concerned about the welfare of his staff, who were exhausted. Psychologists were brought into the wards to counsel staff each week. After many months reflecting on the Delta wave, what stayed with him most, he said, was just how misled people were by hardline conspiracy theories.

'These were ordinary people, and pre-pandemic, they were just good, decent, hardworking people, and somehow, during the pandemic, they became infected with stupidity.' French likened it to Dietrich Bonhoeffer's theory of stupidity, which originated during the Nazi movement in World War II. Bonhoeffer, a theologian, had tried to understand how people could suddenly believe or do awful things. 'It's not a question of intelligence, because intelligent people can be stupid,' French said. 'But during the pandemic, people were basically fed information, often via automated news feeds, on various web-based platforms, and then believed in it. Ultimately, it caused them and their families quite significant distress.'

If it had not been for the lockdowns, New South Wales and Victoria would have run out of hospital beds during the Delta wave. At its peak, there were more than 1,200 patients in New South Wales hospitals and 800 in Victoria, equal to about three or four very large hospitals. To ration the available beds for many months in 2021, only urgent surgery for the sickest people at risk of imminent death was permitted.

The separation of the dying from their loved ones was perhaps the cruelest part of the pandemic. From the beginning, Warrillow said the Austin Hospital took a pragmatic approach to end-of-life care. Wherever it was possible and safe, they allowed a dying person to be with a loved one. Relatives were ushered to the bedside, swathed in plastic, masked and gowned behind thick Perspex visors, to be close to the dying person in their final moments. For those who could not be there in person, nurses held iPads and iPhones to families to see their loved one taking their final breaths. 'We always found ways that were safe for somebody to be there with them when there was genuine end-of-life care and someone was not going to survive,' Warrillow said. 'We never wanted anyone to die alone.'

CHAPTER SEVENTEEN

The lockdown effect

From the doorway of her grocery store in the back streets of Armadale, Louise Graham watched the world grind to a halt during the coronavirus lockdowns. The once-bustling High Street in Melbourne's south-eastern suburbs was deserted, robbed of its colour and joy. As the months passed, shop owners cleared out their window displays, emptied their stores, and vacated them. 'It was just completely dead,' the mother-of-four said. 'I remember feeling so sad. People spent years building their business, and they just couldn't pay their rent anymore.' The caterer lost almost half her income overnight as events were shut down across the city.

While Graham's shop, called The Little Grocer, was permitted to stay open during the lockdowns, many regular customers were so fearful of catching the virus that they refused to come inside. The shelves were stacked all the way to the ceiling, overflowing with local produce, homemade meals, and baked goods. She set up a big trestle table on the street, stacking it with food and freshly baked bread. The orders were flooding in from her older customers, who began requesting takeaway meals every night because they were terrified of catching the virus at the supermarket. She rotated a menu of curries, tomato and basil tarts, and her famous chicken-and-leek pies, which she dropped outside their doors.

During the lockdown months, she became a confidante to people who wandered into her store in search of the human contact snatched away by the pandemic. 'Sometimes I was the only other person they had seen that day or that week, and they could whinge to me, and I could have a whinge back as well,' she said. 'I felt like we were all in solidarity. We were all upset about the same things.'

Graham comforted a grief-stricken woman who had miscarried. She cooked meals for another woman to take to the family of her best friend who had taken her own life, leaving behind a baby and a husband. People sometimes burst into tears at her store when she asked them how they were.

She saw the best of humanity and the worst of it during Melbourne's lockdown. 'A couple of times, people were screaming at each other in the shop if somebody wasn't wearing a mask or they were standing too close … that was such a weird thing. But there were also people who were wonderful and selfless, and looked out for each other during a really tough time.'

By early 2021, Graham could no longer afford her rent, becoming one of many small businesses in Melbourne forced to permanently close during the pandemic.

The same year, a deputy secretary at the federal Treasury, Luke Yeaman, estimated that for every day that Melbourne was locked down in August and September, an average of 1,200 people lost their jobs, and $100 million in economic activity was forgone. By early 2023, the lockdowns were over, but demand for food banks was higher in Australia than it had been during the height of the pandemic. Two-thirds of people on income support were eating less or skipping meals as they grappled with rental stress. Australian families were experiencing the steepest cost-of-living increases in decades, driven in part by higher mortgage costs.

Researchers across the world continue to investigate the implications of the unique stresses triggered by the pandemic and the lockdowns. The coronavirus pandemic created many conditions that can trigger psychological distress: unexpected disruptions to people's employment, social isolation, and millions bereaved. In Australia, many groups suffered disproportionately due to the pandemic — perhaps none more so than young people. Although they were the least likely group to become sick from coronavirus, young people and children were disproportionately affected by the biggest disruption to education in modern history. When coronavirus began to sweep across the country in March 2020, schools in every Australian state and across the world shuttered their doors. Remote instruction effectively became a national policy during major outbreaks. In Victoria, children and teenagers missed around 200 days of face-to-face learning in 2020 and 2021, out of a usual total of about 360.

Louise Graham's oldest daughter, Grace, was in her final year of school in 2020. The pandemic robbed her of key milestones: a valedictory dinner and final assemblies. 'As a mum, I still get really upset about that,' Graham said, her voice cracking with emotion. Through months of remote learning, Graham's teenage children were scattered across the house, their schoolbooks and laptops stacked on desks in the study, living room, and bedrooms. 'It was a stressful time. You were just trying to get them to stay focused and motivated at home. As time went on, that got harder and harder.'

But it was Graham's daughter Harriet, who had been diagnosed with autism, anxiety, and attention deficit hyperactivity disorder, who suffered most during the months of remote learning. Harriet, who was in year eight during the lockdowns of 2020, spent hours a day in her bedroom alone with her laptop. She stopped communicating with friends and walking her dog, the activity she had loved doing most.

'Not being at school was terrible for her,' the mother-of-four said. 'She was just starting to settle in and make friends, and for the first time in a long time she seemed happy, and then everything was just shut down and it all fell apart.'

It was almost as if coming out of lockdown was harder for Harriet, whose anxiety about returning to the classroom became so severe that she started vomiting on the way to school. The 16-year-old is now one of a growing number of teenagers who have become school refusers. Experts told *The Age* that the issue was growing at an alarming rate in Australia, and that schools lacked the resources to overcome the worsening problem, which principals said had been supercharged by Covid-19. The phenomenon is distinct from truancy, in that it is driven by a high level of anxiety and distress about attending school. In Victoria, the rate of school refusal grew by 50 per cent in the three years to 2021, according to a submission made by the state government to a Senate inquiry examining the national trend. The submission revealed that almost 12,000 students in government schools were officially absent in the second year of the pandemic.

Many parents, like Graham, struggled to find support for their children when specialist clinics across Melbourne became booked out, and doctors also closed their books as they dealt with a record rise in children being diagnosed with complex behavioural and mental health problems.

Psychiatrist and former Australian of the Year Patrick McGorry, the executive director of Orygen Youth Health, a Melbourne-based research, policy, and education organisation that specialises in youth mental health, does not dispute that strong public health measures were needed in Victoria before vaccines were deployed, to slow the spread of the virus. However, he said that while governments pulled out all stops and spared no expense to protect the lives of older people at risk of death and serious disease, they failed to put in any plan to support young people, who faced minimal risks but bore the brunt of containment measures.

'This is not about being ageist, or saying older people aren't equally valuable and that we shouldn't have done everything we could to help them and save their lives,' McGorry said. 'Of course older people are valuable. But why did we do that, and we did nothing to help young people? As usual, it is the young people that are not equally valued.

They basically mortgaged the whole country to save the lives of the older people without a thought or plan in place for what happened to young people during the pandemic and the aftermath.'

Soon after the pandemic was declared, University of Melbourne paediatrician Professor Fiona Russell and child health researchers from the Murdoch Children's Research Institute began to do a weekly analysis, investigating the latest global evidence of the implications of coronavirus for children. What was clear to them from early 2020 was that Victorian school closures and a lack of face-to-face social welfare services were fuelling a sharp rise in stress among families. Some of these distressed families were arriving at hospital emergency departments because everything else was closed, or support services had gone online. Doctors began to observe concerning trends, including more babies being hospitalised with poor growth because first-time mothers were struggling to feed them to the point that they were malnourished or failing to thrive.

The worst impacts were being carried by families who relied on support from social services, including those where children were neglected or abused, or had parents with alcohol and drug addictions. A Commission for Children and Young People's annual report found two children in Victoria died after child protection services reduced face-to-face visits and services due to Covid-19 restrictions. 'Everything just went behind doors,' Russell said. 'That was extremely disturbing for paediatricians from mid-2020, and it was a profound concern.'

During Melbourne's second lockdown in 2020, Victoria's Bacchus Marsh Grammar School principal Andrew Neal found his school, which is one of the biggest in the state, suddenly in no man's land. The school, which has more than 3,000 students from prep to year 12, and more than 200 staff, was located just outside Melbourne's 'ring of steel', a barrier enforced by the government to protect regional Victoria from Melbourne's continuing outbreaks. Before the school decided to divert to remote learning, Neal was flooded with 'long epistles' from locals in Bacchus Marsh accusing him of bringing the virus into the town, which was situated mid-way between Melbourne and Ballarat, by allowing busloads of children to attend school.

'It was almost medieval hysteria over those two years,' Neal said. 'They thought I should be basically on the barricades stopping them from coming in.' But it wasn't just the locals who were up in arms. 'There were parents on the fringes at either end,' Neal recalled. 'We had the fringe that wanted us to close down and never reopen. Then there were the parents in the other direction who thought it was all hokum and wanted us back at school every waking moment.'

Ultimately, the school decided to go online for much of 2020 to protect staff and students from the virus. Neal said that he and his staff 'basically invented' what remote schooling looked like within a week. 'A lot of people assumed there was some giant rulebook handed out where you just flick to page 500 and there was the answer, but that didn't exist,' Neale said. 'There were certainly no instructions from the government. We just cobbled something together, and hoped it would work.'

Initially, Neal said the students loved being able to roll out of bed and learn from their bedrooms or living rooms on laptops and iPads through Zoom. But as the lockdowns continued into mid-2021, teenage students, in particular, began to disengage. Teachers and parents burned out. 'There were teenage kids who did not want to be seen on a screen, and other kids finding it increasingly hard to get out of bed,' Neale said. 'We were also relying on technology that wasn't necessarily 100 per cent, so it was very, very difficult. The notion that productivity increased in remote learning was a complete fallacy.'

Neal said there was real grief about the children who missed their first year of prep and the year 12 students who were robbed of key adolescent milestones such as socials and formals. 'I had a mother in tears in my office. She was just devastated that her daughter was cheated out of her first year in prep,' Neal said.

The school would find itself at the centre of a coronavirus cluster in 2021. Neal said he barely slept during that outbreak. Each day, he would spend hours on the phone to about 20 staff and students infected. 'Some of them got very, very sick, and one of our teachers came very close to dying after ending up in the ICU,' Neal said.

When students returned to the classroom in late 2021, Neale observed a distinct lack of socialisation. There were more 'petty arguments' among both primary school pupils and early-year high school students in the classrooms. 'What it really came down to was just this incapacity for some of the kids to deal with the reality of 30 different individuals in a classroom,' he said. Among the older students, the implications of the pandemic manifested themselves in what Neal described as a deep and pronounced adolescent malaise. Their appetite for learning and engaging socially with their peers was diminished. There was also a level of anxiety disorders and increase in school-refuser rates beyond anything he had observed in his decades-long career. 'It was quite striking, really,' Neal said.

Another effect of Victoria's response to the pandemic was the number of children who stopped eating. Soon after Melbourne's second lockdown began, emergency departments reported a dramatic rise in children coming in with eating disorders. Weekly presentations more than doubled, and the Royal Children's Hospital reported a surge of seriously ill kids who had starved themselves to the point where they needed to be admitted into the specialist eating-disorder ward.

Jo Foggo's 14-year-old daughter was one of the teenagers who developed anorexia during the pandemic in Melbourne. It seemed to sneak up on the family. At first, the teenager was quietly skipping meals when her parents weren't around. Her weight plunged as her family battled to get the right specialist support. Psychologists told them they had waiting lists that were six months long, or that their books were closed. Appointments were cancelled. At home, the teenager lay on the ground, screaming and refusing any food. Eventually, Foggo's daughter became so unwell that she needed to be hospitalised. 'She was clasping at her heart,' recalled Foggo. 'I said, "This is not right."' When the teenager was admitted to the eating-disorder ward, she had the lowest body mass index that the local youth mental health service had seen in five years.

After a 12-day stay, when she regained just enough weight to be considered medically stable, her daughter was abruptly discharged one afternoon, Foggo said. During her stint on the ward, she had not been provided with any mental health support. There was no offer for help in the home, with Foggo instead given the crushing task of supervising meals to keep her daughter alive.

There were many stories like this. Child and youth psychiatrist Dr Anthony Gallagher said there was also a downward trend in the age of the young people with eating disorders. Children as young as eight or nine needed treatment. These desperately ill kids and their parents then discovered that there was no help in their moment of crisis, or it was inadequate. There were too few specialists, and the hospitals often took only the most gravely ill—those so sick that their internal organs were strained, and who were at risk of dying.

Clinical psychologist Dr Linsey Atkins, who specialises in treating children with severe eating disorders, was shocked by how quickly her young patients deteriorated at the beginning of the pandemic. By May 2020, she said, 'Most of the kids on my books were suicidal, and that's not something that I had experienced previously.' By 2023, there was a young girl in Melbourne who had been readmitted to hospital for anorexia more than 30 times.

Anorexia has the highest death rate of any psychiatric disorder. It eats away at children, but also at the very foundation of their families: scarring siblings, destroying marriages, and crippling parents financially. Lockdowns and the pandemic increased the risk factors for disordered eating: matters such as social isolation, disruption to routines, and heightened anxiety. The rise in disordered eating among young people has become a global pandemic phenomenon, with similar trends reported in Canada and the US.

As the months dragged on, Fiona Russell and her colleagues were determined to get schools reopened because it was a safety net for children, particularly those living in abusive households. In the first year of the pandemic, the paediatrician led a study of Covid-19 school closures with a group of colleagues from the Murdoch Children's Research Institute. Their report found that of a million enrolled students in Victoria, only 337 or 0.03 per cent had a coronavirus infection linked to a school outbreak in 2020. Ultimately, their study suggested that schools should have remained open when there were less transmissible variants circulating before Delta emerged.

Russell said that, pre-Delta, the immunology showed that children were able to clear the virus faster, and therefore were less likely to transmit it. 'What we found in all our research was that schools reflected transmission in the community, but they did not drive it.' Russell and her colleagues believed that outbreaks could be controlled by testing, quarantining, and contact tracing, arguing that schools should only be closed 'as a last resort'. Rather than the government imposing blanket closures during outbreaks, the researchers recommended that a staged mitigation strategy be adopted, or a traffic-light system, allowing schools in Australia to stay open, and children and staff to be kept safe through measures such as physical distancing, the wearing of masks, and the adoption of class bubbles.

They presented their findings to the Australian Health Protection Principal Committee and the World Health Organisation. But, months later, there was still no national plan about how to manage schools during the pandemic. Experts, including Russell and principals such as Andrew Neal, began to push for teachers and school support staff to be prioritised for vaccinations to get children back in the classroom. Neal remembered publicly offering to inoculate his own staff, just to get the school open quicker.

Russell's view was that Australian children were an afterthought in coronavirus policies. 'Children were seen primarily as "vectors" rather than individuals with unique social and developmental needs,' she said.

The legacy of what Russell refers to as prolonged 'toxic stress' on children remains unknown. 'Many children will be fine,' she said. 'But there will be another group that won't be. The consequences will change the trajectory of their entire life for the worse. We have no idea how many that will be, so in a sense this has been one giant experiment.' She said while closing schools in response to outbreaks early in the pandemic in 2020 was justified, by September 2020 it was clearly known that coronavirus wasn't a major problem for children. 'On a grand scale, it was very clear the indirect effects were worse than the direct effects,' Russell said. 'The indirect effects on children were enormous. But in this pandemic, the needs of children were pretty much ignored.'

As coronavirus spread globally, countries across the world grappled with how to manage the implications for children who were locked out of their schools. Singapore reopened its schools in mid-2021 when 70 per cent of adults had received one vaccine dose. Denmark started sending children back to school in February 2021, with just 4 per cent vaccine coverage among adults, moving children into outdoor classrooms and even to cemeteries. In Spain, classrooms were moved to the open air of the beaches to reduce the risk of outbreaks. Other countries invested in improving air filtration and outdoor classrooms. 'The real question is why didn't Australia do what other countries were doing,' Russell said.

A former chair of the World Health Organisation's Global Outbreak Alert and Response Network, Professor Dale Fisher, said one of the striking features of the pandemic in Australia was its often binary approach to decision-making, particularly around school closures. 'It was either you open schools, or you close them all,' the Australian-born infectious disease expert at the National University of Singapore said. 'Now, I would say that's not ideal, and you can be a lot more innovative than that. Where was the middle ground?'

In Singapore, Fisher said there was a blended learning model: when cases were high, children could go to school for a few days and then learn remotely for the rest of the week. Masks were mandated indoors for children over five, and desks were spread out. Rather than a Covid-zero policy, the country had an aggressive containment strategy, which kept coronavirus cases low. It allowed people to move more freely, but a strict baseline of restrictions remained in place for years. The country only lifted mandatory mask-wearing on public transport in 2023.

Fisher believed that Australia may have avoided some lockdowns had it enforced a moderate baseline of rules nationally, irrespective of whether there were outbreaks. While this would have meant taking more unpopular political decisions, such as continuing bans on mass gatherings and sporting matches, Fisher believes it could have avoided wild swings in Victoria between harsh lockdowns followed by minimal and decreasing restrictions when no local cases were being detected.

'Covid-zero was not, in my view, ever a good long-term plan,' he said. 'There was this pressure in Australia that as soon as you got back to zero, things could be normal again, and that is just not how a pandemic works.'

When asked about the school closures, Victoria's chief health officer, Brett Sutton, expressed regret that Australia had not acted faster in March 2020 to close its borders, which he believes could have avoided the initial two months of remote learning. But he strongly disputes the idea that further school closures were not necessary in his state. 'I do challenge the notion that they were not required at all, or that transmission was not substantial amongst children, or was not substantial amongst schools,' Sutton said. 'It's pretty clear, especially from the serosurveys [used to detect the spread in the community] that children were infected at some of the highest rates amongst the entire population, and therefore schools were a significant driver.'

Sutton said that because classrooms were indoors, more than a million children would have been in a high-risk indoor environment for hours each day, and this would have inevitably driven up community transmission. He said that had Victoria not been striving to get transmission back down to zero, school closures would have been considered very differently. Mitigations such as mask-wearing, ventilation, and HEPA filters could have been used more widely. 'But when you're trying to get back to zero transmission because you've got a completely unvaccinated population, then in a Covid-zero strategy … you have to do what's required in schools, and that means remote learning as part of that response,' Sutton said. Mass school closures became one of the most controversial matters during the pandemic, as infectious disease paediatricians went head-to-head with the Victorian government, warning that Victoria was sacrificing the health of children for the sake of the elderly by keeping schools closed.

Victoria's former deputy chief health officer, Professor Allen Cheng, said that, with the benefit of hindsight, the government might have sought to keep schools open more, especially in 2020. But he said that, given Victoria's Covid-zero mindset, the focus was on controlling and eliminating every last case. 'Every time we'd open a school there would be another outbreak, so it was very difficult to do,' Cheng said. 'If we had our time again, we would try to push schools to do their contact tracing themselves. But people weren't as familiar with all those concepts, so it was really difficult back then.'

In the first year of the pandemic, Professor Patrick McGorry presented to the state government a sobering insight into what the pandemic could mean for the mental health of Victorian teenagers and young adults, according to a report by journalist Chip Le Grand. McGorry warned that as many as 370,000 additional Victorians, including 82,000 between the ages of 12 and 25, might experience mental health disorders. This prediction was based on modelling conducted by Orygen's health economist Matthew Hamilton. The modelling showed that the greatest risk to young people was not the virus, but damage to their mental health caused by disengagement and isolation from school, work, and friends, and the subsequent loss of employment prospects. This shadow pandemic, as McGorry calls it, is predicted to peak in the years to come after coronavirus has disappeared from the headlines.

During Victoria's lockdowns of 2020 and 2021, there was a sharp rise in the number of teenagers and young people seeking emergency care. One report by the Victorian Agency for Health Information revealed a 72 per cent increase in the number of serious self-harm and suicidal-ideation presentations in hospital emergency departments among under-18s during the final lockdown in 2020. McGorry said that the most common pattern observed by physicians was a rise in young women presenting with a 'nasty combination of anxiety, depression, self-harm cutting, and eating disorders'.

Research from the University of New South Wales also showed an 82 per cent increase in child and adolescent inpatient hospital admissions nationally for self-harm between March 2020 and December 2021. While those presentations dropped slightly after restrictions eased, the study found they remained higher than pre-pandemic levels.

In 2022, the national survey of mental health, which is conducted every 15 years, found a 50 per cent rise in mental health problems in young people. Two in five young Australians were found have a mental illness and to need support. But McGorry said that systemic problems and chronic underfunding had long plagued Victoria's mental health sector before coronavirus came along.

McGorry was in contact with many politicians who raised concerns about lockdowns and the impacts they were having on young people. He recalled a concerned Scott Morrison calling him late one night in 2020 asking, 'What do I do?' McGorry said that, to the prime minister's credit, he heeded the advice McGorry gave him, immediately increasing funding to Headspace, a national youth mental health foundation, so that support workers could visit young people in their homes.

McGorry believes that Victorian officials and politicians, most notably health minister Martin Foley and premier Daniel Andrews, were also genuinely concerned about the welfare of young people. He said that Foley acted by increasing funding for digital mental health care programs for young people. 'But, unfortunately, these were isolated incidents,' McGorry said. 'Most of the mental health responses were superficial.'

The royal commission into Victoria's mental health system resulted in hundreds of millions of dollars being allocated to rebuild the mental health sector. But McGorry said that, during the height of the pandemic, the state government suffered from a 'degree of tunnel vision' and was too overwhelmed in dealing with coronavirus in the state's hospitals to do anything about mental health that would have any serious effect.

When Australia decided to close schools, the national children's commissioner, Anne Hollonds, said that nobody really considered the needs of children. 'I was pretty horrified at some of the things that went on,' she said. 'Children were invisible, even though the impacts of things like school closures were huge and life-changing for them.' Hollonds, who has travelled around Australia investigating the implications of Covid for children, said she had heard distressing accounts from parents of suicidal children under the age of 12 who were sent away from overwhelmed public hospitals and told to find a private psychiatrist.

'If you can't get a suicidal child into a public health environment urgently, there is something seriously wrong with our system,' she said. 'What was completely invisible during the pandemic were the children living in poverty and disadvantage, and families with kids with disabilities. There were some families in Melbourne's public housing towers where there were six children trying to be home-schooled with one laptop. When you look back, it's just terrible what happened.'

Like Fiona Russell, Hollonds remained concerned about a potentially lost generation of children, who, at a very critical stage of their development, did not get the support they needed. Some never returned to schools when lockdowns ended. 'Throughout the pandemic, there was just nobody sitting at that top level who was advocating for the needs of children,' said Hollonds, who has previously called for Australia to appoint a national children's minister. 'It is something that must never happen again in a crisis.'

She said the greatest lesson from the pandemic was that schools

were much more than a place of academic learning. Among Hollonds'
most scathing criticisms was the fact that more than two years passed
without a national pandemic framework being adopted for children
and schools. Hollonds, who lives in Sydney, recalled being 'horrified and appalled' when pubs and restaurants were reopened in New
South Wales before students were allowed to return to the classroom
following the deadly Delta wave of 2021.

The psychologist was a key contributor to *Fault Lines: an independent review into Australia's response to Covid-19*, led by former
public servant and chancellor of Western Sydney University Peter
Shergold, which analysed hundreds of submissions and consultations
with health experts, economists, welfare groups, and businesses. The
report argued that while school closures had been justified at the start
of the pandemic, governments departed from the nation's pandemic
planning and health advice by shutting all classes for entire school
terms in 2020 and 2021. It also found that the excessive use of lockdowns had failed to protect the old, had disregarded the young, and
had abandoned some of the nation's most disadvantaged communities. Frontline workers, women, children, aged-care residents,
people with disabilities, ethnic communities, international students,
expatriates, and those already experiencing relative socio-economic
disadvantage bore the brunt of the pandemic, the review found. 'Left
unchecked, the recovery threatens to be just as unequal.'

During lockdowns, women overwhelmingly bore the brunt of all the
domestic duties and home-schooling. The toll of this was laid bare
when Victorian women sought mental health support at record levels
in 2020 and 2021. Professor Jayashri Kulkarni, who runs the Alfred
Hospital women's mental health clinic in Melbourne, said the data
collected globally clearly showed that women of all ages around the
world struggled more with depression, anxiety, eating disorders, and
post-traumatic stress due to the impacts of the pandemic.

It was during Melbourne's second wave and the subsequent

lockdowns of 2021 that Kulkarni observed an escalation in demand she had never experienced before in her decades-long career. 'The clinic just absolutely exploded in terms of the numbers of people wanting help,' she said. 'The acuity was extraordinary. There were really horrible, awful situations, where women were calling me from their bathroom or toilet, extremely distressed, because that was the only place that they could actually have some privacy or call safely and have a consultation.' The professor of psychiatry at Monash University treated a sharp rise in women with self-harm injuries and suicidal ideation, an increase in home-schooling mothers who had turned to alcohol to cope, and a significant cohort of people who had never experienced mental health problems before Covid-19.

For younger women, it was the psychological consequences of social isolation or living alone that turned a mild bout of anxiety or depression into a deep depression or complex anxiety disorder. For women in their 30s, 40s, and 50s, the stress of home-schooling on top of other duties, such as caring for elderly parents or relatives, and the economic stress of the pandemic, were all contributing factors that sparked a tidal wave in mental health problems.

'Women were largely responsible for bearing, caring, rearing, and home-schooling of children,' she said. 'It was a huge role. They also make up a significant portion of the casual labour force, so as the economic downturn occurred they presented with stresses around joblessness and money. They lost their jobs in greater numbers than men.' Kulkarni said that home-schooling also contributed to women leaving the workplace to carry the burden, adding that one unknown is the lasting effects of two years of prolonged isolation and the loneliness that came with it.

The coronavirus lockdown also put a strain on couples, with some Australian family therapists and lawyers noting a jump in people seeking counselling or filing for a divorce. A study on the impacts of Covid-19 by Relationships Australia found that 42 per cent of people had experienced a negative change in their relationship with their partner in 2020. Rates of family violence also rose during the pandemic in Australia, a phenomenon documented globally during lockdowns. The United Nations called the situation a 'shadow pandemic' in a 2021 report about domestic violence in 13 nations in Africa, Asia, South America, Eastern Europe, and the Balkans. Research reported in the *American Journal of Emergency Medicine* suggested that domestic violence cases increased by 25 to 33 percent globally.

In July 2020, a separate survey by the Australian Institute of Criminology revealed that about 10 per cent of Australian women in a relationship who were surveyed for the study had reported experiencing domestic violence during the early months of the pandemic. Two-thirds of the women said the attacks started or became worse during the pandemic, while Full Stop Australia, a support service for sexual assault and family violence, reported a 26 per cent increase in calls during the early years of the pandemic.

Kulkarni said this was the tip of the iceberg, noting that many women were unable to call safely while they were compelled to stay home with their abuser. 'The increased level of violence towards women from their partners in lockdowns was obvious in retrospect,' Kulkarni said. 'If she's locked down with somebody who's been abusive, then all hell is going to break loose when she can't get out.' The director of services at Berry Street child and family services, Jenny McNaughton, said one of the most concerning aspects of the pandemic was the trend in men becoming violent for the first time — something that she attributes in part to the stress of the pandemic. In the early days, crucial outreach programs went online. 'There was a real lack of eyes on vulnerable families. There wasn't the teacher picking up warning signs in the kids, or the support worker noticing things about women,' she said. 'Any chance of mediation or early intervention into the problem just didn't happen.'

Patrick McGorry wrote in 2023 that a range of modelling has predicted a substantial rise in mental ill-health and suicide risk in the aftermath of the pandemic. There are socio-economic forces that ebb and flow, and that influence the momentum for suicide in a population. This has been known for more than 100 years. He said that the best examples are that during wartime and times of external threat—perhaps including pandemics—suicide rates fall as communities mobilise to weather a crisis, and after the threat passes, and especially during times of economic stress, they rise. In 2022, Victoria recorded its highest number of annual suicides since the coroner's court started collecting suicide data in 2000. In 2022, there were 756 suicides in Victoria, a 9 per cent increase compared with 2021. From January to July, the monthly number of suicides was consistent with previous years, at approximately 58 suicides a month. From August to December, the number increased to an average of 65 a month. The coroner's court warned that it 'considers that the higher numbers during August to December 2022 might signal an emerging trend'.

The most substantial increase in suicides was seen in the 65 years-and-older cohort, with a 32 per cent rise from 2021 to 2022. There was a 21 per cent increase among people aged 45 to 54, an 8 per cent increase among males, and a 12 per cent increase among females. There has also been a rise in New South Wales, with a suspected 885 suicide deaths reported in 2022, compared with 818 over the same period the year before. Access to expert mental health care and even primary care has become much more difficult post-pandemic. Whether this rise in suicides is occurring in other states, which had fewer coronavirus restrictions, is not yet clear. Victoria and New South Wales are the only states that release monthly data on suicides. Other states and territories report their data to a national database, and the public release of this information can often lag for more than a year.

While demand for mental health support remains immense, there are early positive signs of a reprieve. Australian Health and Welfare institute data at the end of 2022 showed a 6 per cent decrease in demand for such support compared to 2021. At Bacchus Marsh Grammar, the slow march to emotional recovery has begun. Principal Andrew Neal said the school had embraced what he called 'old-fashioned house activities' aimed at getting students to fully engage with school through activities they love. Games, drama classes, and sports have all been increased. 'These are activities where they can follow their passions, and they have to get out and talk to people, and mix with their peers or work together,' he said. The principal said there was no doubt that students had yet to fully catch up academically, but he remained 'extremely optimistic' that most students would bounce back both emotionally and intellectually.

'The notion of it happening within months is what people really need to get out of their minds,' Neal said. 'Kids are very resilient, and as long as we keep supporting them, they will come out of this. But just as Covid has taken two to three years out of our lives, it will take two to three years to get out of it.'

CHAPTER EIGHTEEN

When coronavirus hit the Top End

When coronavirus crept into the tiny Aboriginal community of Binjari, 320 kilometres south of Darwin, the fear was palpable. For almost two years, the Northern Territory government and its health officials had kept the disease out of remote Aboriginal communities. But by 20 November 2021 the virus had seeped into the outback and across the vast deserts. 'It really sent shockwaves through the community,' said the Wurli-Wurlinjang Health Services chief executive, Peter Gazey, who helped lead the emergency response in Binjari. 'Even at that time, it was thought if it got into the community, it would kill a lot of people because of the death rates elsewhere.'

For almost two weeks, Binjari was in lockdown. Floodlights were installed at the outskirts of the tiny town where about 200 Wardaman and Jawoyn people lived. The lights blazed through the night, as a warning to anyone trying to escape the lockdown—shining into the windows of homes, keeping residents awake. Each evening, noisy and slow-flying drones, which sounded like a scourge of mosquitoes, circled dark skies, checking that residents were obeying the stay-at-home orders. In the daytime, the tight-knit community, which is usually lively and social, was eerily quiet. 'People were staying in their own yards, in their own houses, and for the community, that's really unusual,' Gazey said. 'They are always moving around and visiting each other multiple times in a day. Then, all of a sudden, the kids have to stay home, and nobody is allowed out.'

Wardaman woman Olivia Raymond described some of the community being just as frightened of the harsh lockdown measures as they were of the virus itself. 'There was police here walking around the community, and the police over there on the oval, watching over, making us feel like … [it was] an invasion,' she told *Guardian Australia* reporters Lorena Allam and Isabella Moore in June 2022. 'It was like in a movie or something … even though there were a lot of police along the main road. I think there were about five people who wanted to run away that night, because they couldn't stand it.' More than a year later, Binjari local Billy Maroney said the outbreak remained 'one of the worst things' he had ever experienced. 'I think everybody was in for a bit of a shock for a long time that it could happen like this to a remote community like ours,' he told the ABC.

The worst-case scenarios mapped out at the beginning of the pandemic response showed potentially catastrophic effects on Aboriginal communities if the virus were to land in remote parts of the country. Aboriginal Australians made up one in every four Territorians. They have long endured the worst health outcomes of any population nationally, dying on average almost a decade before non-Indigenous Australians.

In the early days of the pandemic, there were fears that coronavirus could mirror the 2009 swine flu outbreak for Aboriginal Australians, when chronic disease and geographical isolation led to devastating outcomes. The swine flu hospitalisation rate was 12 times greater than for non-Indigenous people, and despite only making up less than 4 per cent of the population, they suffered a death rate six times higher than the national average, and accounted for more than 10 per cent of all infections. Scott Morrison, Australia's prime minister, said he had worried it was going to 'wipe out' entire Indigenous populations across the country, especially in remote areas. 'We're talking about the impact of disease like in 1789; that's what we were fearful of.'

When coronavirus eventually made its way to Binjari, police quickly set up a roadblock at the town turn-off, 18 kilometres south-west of Katherine, and the Australian Defence Force was called in to deliver food and to transport Covid-infected patients. The pandemic measures implemented in the Binjari outbreak were among the toughest in Australia, and certainly stricter than restrictions experienced by any other town in the Northern Territory. Gazey said that the health response worked well, at first, reflecting the deep roots and trust built over many years between local health authorities and the remote Aboriginal community. But soon the virus began spreading so quickly that it was impossible for people to isolate themselves from other people in their home. 'The problems were the houses in Binjari,' Gazey explained to *Guardian Australia*. 'Some of them, because people were visiting, had up to 20 people in one house, so there was no way they could isolate and stop the spread.' More than 200 people from Binjari and nearby Katherine would be taken to the Howard Springs quarantine centre, three hours away, where they stayed in self-contained cabins, spaced out in rows.

Most houses in Binjari are run-down and overcrowded. Almost all the properties are in need of urgent essential repairs, with the outbreak exposing the dire conditions of those living there. A public-announcement system was used to blare out house numbers from the nearby Binjari Health Centre, prompting the entire household to come and be tested at the clinic. It was an extraordinarily effective program, Gazey said, ensuring social distancing and also offering a reprieve to the healthcare workers responding to the crisis. Initially, they were saturated in sweat under their personal protective equipment after spending more than 12 hours a day in the sweltering desert heat going from house to house. Gazey said that contact tracing was made easy by the closeness of the community and their desire to protect each other. Their actions, the work of Aboriginal leaders, and local healthcare workers on the ground became a model for how to curtail a potentially disastrous outbreak and protect a high-risk community.

However, as the virus spread in Binjari, there was an explosion of misinformation and conspiracy theories. Anti-vaccination videos—in which people claimed that residents were being forcibly removed from their homes by the army, children were being taken from the parents, and others were being vaccinated against their will—began to go viral on Facebook and Instagram. The videos were flooding in from all over the world, including from as far away as North America and the United Kingdom.

The usually calm Northern Territory chief minister, Michael Gunner, lost his cool during a press conference over the 'crazy rumours' being circulated. 'There are ridiculous, untrue rumours about the Australian Defence Force's involvement. As we all know, they aren't carrying weapons—they are carrying fresh food for people,' Gunner told a media briefing on 25 November 2021 providing an update on the outbreak. 'Ninety-nine-point-nine-nine per cent of the BS [bullshit] that is flying around on the internet about the territory is coming from flogs outside the territory—mostly America, Canada, and the UK. If anybody thinks that we are going to be distracted or intimidated by tinfoil-hat–wearing tossers, sitting in their parents' basements in Florida, then you do not know us territorians.'

Binjari elders issued a public statement condemning the rumours as false. 'We are in lockdown because we're in the biggest fight of our lives. We're trying to keep safe,' they wrote. 'We're trying to do the right thing by the community and Katherine. We don't appreciate outside people making comments that are untrue. People on social media saying that our people are being mistreated need to realise their comments are hurting the very people they claim to care about.'

A 78-year-old woman and Binjari elder became the first person in the Northern Territory to die of coronavirus. Instead of being by her bedside in hospital, the woman's family were at the Howard Springs quarantine facility. She was the only Binjari resident to die in the outbreak, though many others were hospitalised. Dozens of infections cropped up in the tiny desert communities of Robinson River and Rockhole, sparking widespread testing, lockdowns, and temporary mask mandates. Covid fragments would be detected in wastewater as far away as 900 kilometres north-west of Alice Springs. When the outbreak hit, vaccination rates were dangerously low in some Indigenous communities.

The cluster of about 50 cases would be traced back to a 21-year-old woman with Covid who illegally entered the Northern Territory after contracting the virus in Victoria and lying on her border entry form. She infected a man in Darwin before the virus spread to Katherine, and then to the Aboriginal communities of Robinson River, Binjari, Rockhole, and Lajamanu. Binjari would experience the harshest restrictions, staying in lockdown for almost two weeks.

While many Indigenous Australians were eager to get the vaccine when the virus began spreading in their communities, Gazey said third and fourth booster doses, critical in protecting against more infectious variants of the disease, plummeted in the aftermath. Worryingly, childhood immunisations have also dropped off. There has been a marked pandemic-fuelled increase in other deadly diseases among Indigenous Australians, the consequences of which are yet to be fully understood. Wurli-Wurlinjang Health Services has about 5,000 clients, many of whom have chronic health conditions such as diabetes, elevating their risk of severe disease from Covid.

'You've got things like diabetes not being attended to. People's blood sugars are higher, there have been more hospitalisations and treatment because of that. With kidney disease, we've found people are now more end-stage,' Gazey said. 'There's been a marked increase or decline in people's conditions.' The reasons why are multifactorial, Gazey said. Medical treatment has never ceased in Binjari, but some people have delayed seeking it, or have struggled to secure appointments with specialists due to government-enforced travel restrictions.

The Northern Territory emerged from the chaos of the first two years of the pandemic having spent a minuscule amount of time in lockdown compared to eastern states such as Victoria and New South

Wales. The vast majority of the 106 coronavirus cases detected in the territory in the first year of the pandemic were at the Howard Springs quarantine facility. It was one of the only places in Australia where there were no reports of community transmission, and in the first year, at least, there were no coronavirus deaths. It was one of Australia's great triumphs—and not just because of Howard Springs—that it did not report a single coronavirus outbreak or breach over the more than two years it welcomed returnees.

The pandemic had started in dramatic fashion for the territory's chief minister, Michael Gunner. On 18 January 2020, while at home with wife, ABC journalist Kristy O'Brien, who was then pregnant with their first son, Hudson, Gunner felt a sharp pain in his chest. Doctors would later tell him he had had a major heart attack, likely caused by a blood clot. He needed three operations, including major surgery in Adelaide, to plug a hole in his heart.

'I was just terrified,' said 46-year-old Gunner, who is the first person born in the Northern Territory to be elected chief minister in the government's history. 'It was serious—it wasn't small. I've learnt that more as time has gone on. There were times at home when I just cried to my wife. Suddenly, you're thinking, *Will I not be here for the kid?* Gunner heeded advice given to him early in his career: 'There's no such thing as a sick politician. When you're in public, you're well.' Under strict doctor's orders, he took two weeks off work; but exactly a fortnight later, he was back door-knocking in Darwin's humid wet season for an impending byelection that had been called after his colleague, Labor politician Ken Vowles, was sacked for publicly criticising the government's economic management.

The Northern Territory's mantra was to 'act hard and fast', and on 21 March 2020 it became the second Australian jurisdiction to announce it would shut its borders to the rest of the country, two days after Tasmania did so. Weeks earlier, Darwin had taken in the country's first 'coronavirus refugees', a decision made following uproar over a federal government decision to send the first tranche of Australian evacuees from China to quarantine for 14 days on Christmas Island, notorious as an offshore prison for asylum seekers.

Gunner counts the deal he struck with the federal government to take in coronavirus evacuees and to quarantine them in Howard Springs as among his proudest moments as leader. The Labor politician said he shared a productive and close working relationship with the Liberal prime minister, Scott Morrison, particularly on matters of protecting remote Aboriginal Australians from the virus. 'I spoke to Scott a lot. I could call him or text him at any time, and he always listened,' Gunner said. 'He did everything he could to help the territory. It was just a genuinely honest and respectful relationship all the way through Covid.'

A Qantas flight carrying 266 weary Australians who had been evacuated from the coronavirus epicentre in Wuhan, China, landed in Darwin on 9 February 2020, the second of two rescue missions. After touching down, the travellers disembarked through the Royal Australian Air Force base, rather than the main airport terminal, and were whisked away to Howard Springs, a disused Manigurr-Ma work camp. There were no antiviral treatments or vaccines available, and about 800 people in China had already succumbed to the virus.

Royal Melbourne Hospital emergency nurse Cherylynn McGurgan was on board the rescue flight that flew from Melbourne to Wuhan and then back to Darwin. The heating was turned off in the darkened plane as children who had been infected with coronavirus battled soaring temperatures. She spent much of the more-than-14-hour flight comforting the feverish children and carefully showing passengers how to safely put on and take off their face masks. 'It was the middle of winter and flu season in China, and we were stripping layers of clothes off these sweating children who were piling onto the plane, and the magnitude of it all hit me,' McGurgan recalled. 'A pandemic hadn't been declared then, but it really dawned on me just how vulnerable we would all be to this virus, and how much work we had to do.'

In the stifling wet-season heat and humidity, dressed head to toe in full personal protective gear as sweat poured off her, the experienced nurse spent weeks setting up medical clinics and caring for people in quarantine at Howard Springs. 'We had a six-month-old baby and a 92-year-old retired doctor that I was taking care of, so it was not only about screening people for the virus, but also all the logistical things like how can we safely get items from the supermarket like baby formula to them,' McGurgan said.

The mission would serve as a crash course of sorts in how to respond to coronavirus, and later would become the catalyst for McGurgan driving the Royal Melbourne Hospital's response to the virus after she helped transform Darwin's Howard Springs quarantine facility. Back in Melbourne, McGurgan would use the lessons learnt in Darwin to help transform the Royal Melbourne Hospital's emergency department, setting up screening clinics that would test tens of thousands of Victorians, and hosting seminars teaching Australian healthcare workers how to safely use personal protective equipment.

But then, after having been exposed to thousands of cases of coronavirus in her job on the frontline of Victoria's severe second wave, McGurgan fell ill while setting up a screening clinic for residents in Melbourne's public housing towers. 'I had never had a headache like it,' she said. 'It felt like somebody had put a metal band around my head, and Goliath was on the other end squeezing to see if he could make two heads out of one.' The virus spread to her joints, leaving her with debilitating neurological symptoms, including persistent headaches and searing pain, that endure years later.

Gunner's first son, Hudson, burst into this strange new world on 9 April 2020. But there was no time for paternity leave. Instead, the doting dad transformed his office at Parliament House into what he dubbed a 'working-dad zone'. He set up a cot in his office, and stuck a sign on the door warning visitors to knock in case the baby was feeding or sleeping. Hudson became known as the 'national cabinet baby'. His name appeared in the meeting minutes. The fair-haired, brown-eyed baby didn't know it, but he was in a position that any journalist in Australia would have dreamt of, witnessing discussions among the most powerful leaders in the country, and some of the most substantial decisions in the nation's history. In between serious deliberations on matters of national importance, Western Australian premier Mark McGowan, a friend and confidant of Gunner's, would often take photos of Hudson cuddled up in Gunner's arms, and send them to him via text.

There were a few close calls in the Northern Territory, including the infamous Granites gold mine outbreak in late June 2021. The mine sits on the Tanami Road, a sprawling, vast red-dirt track connecting Central Australia to Western Australia, some 540 kilometres north-west of Alice Springs. It was from this large hole in the ground between Balgo and Chilla Well in the Tanami desert that Covid spread to four different states. The outbreak, which grew to five cases, sent both Darwin and Alice Springs into their first short, sharp lockdowns.

The head of the Northern Territory's rapid response to coronavirus, Professor Di Stephens, would credit the gold mine's owner's decision to close down the mine at 2.00 am as crucial in preventing a national disaster. 'This single action done at a critical point in time saved the Northern Territory, and probably the country,' she said. But while the outbreak flared from the very remote mine, it had seeded from a far less obscure source: hotel quarantine. Patient zero for the outbreak turned out to be a mine worker who had become infected while in quarantine at a hotel for one night in Brisbane, after travelling to the city from regional Victoria. From Brisbane, the worker flew into the mine on a charter plane. Almost a week later, he was notified of the hotel quarantine leak. The worker then tested positive, and the mine was plunged into lockdown. About 750 workers were sent into immediate quarantine. But by then Covid had already spread. Before anyone knew that Covid was inside the mine, about 900 FIFO workers had flown home across the country.

There is still a hint of frustration about this outbreak when we broach the subject with Gunner. At that time, every state and territory had their own rules around quarantining Australians coming from interstate. The irony is that, had the mine worker arrived in the Northern Territory without having stopped over in Queensland, he would never have been infected with coronavirus to begin with. In fact, he wouldn't even have had to quarantine because, unlike in Queensland, regional Victoria was not considered high risk by the Northern Territory at that time. 'It was a classic situation where I just felt a more practical response which measured risk would have been a better way of dealing with it,' Gunner said. There was also another quick lockdown soon after, stretching from 16 to 19 August in Greater Darwin, after an international arrival, who came from the United States for work purposes, tested positive to the virus, despite quarantining in Sydney before flying to the Top End.

Like so many across the world, Gunner emerged as a changed person from the upheaval of the pandemic. There is a clarity that comes from a brush with death, such as having a heart attack on the precipice of a global pandemic while you're one of the country's leaders. Gunner knew that his career in politics was coming to an end. He was exhausted, but he hung on to lead the Labor Party to victory in the Northern Territory's state election in August 2020, describing it as the only political campaign in history during which a politician did not make a single pre-election promise. 'I said we've got one job to do, and that's to deal with Covid, and we are not going to make promises,' he recalled. 'It was the biggest issue in the world … the biggest issue in the Northern Territory.'

On 29 April 2022, Gunner's second son, Nash, 'a big, happy lad of 3.8 kilograms with very strong lungs and a healthy appetite', arrived in the world. Gunner's heart ached to be at home with his family. Weeks later, he resigned as chief minister, moments after handing down the Northern Territory budget. 'Welcoming little Nash into the world sealed the deal,' he said. 'My head and heart were no longer in it. I wanted to be at home. I'll always be grateful for Covid in a strange way, because it has an amazing capacity to reset all your priorities.'

CHAPTER NINETEEN

RATs

People scoffed at the front page of *The Sydney Morning Herald* on 21 December 2021. 'Absurd,' wrote one reader. 'Clearly implausible,' tutted another. The newspaper's headline warned that new cases of the infectious Omicron strain of Covid could hit 200,000 a day in Australia. It was a number so high that to get there, the country's daily cases would have to climb to more than 40 times the record at the time. It was not surprising that some found it ludicrous. But Australia's chief medical officer, Paul Kelly, did not think it was crazy. The purpose of disease modelling is not to predict the future, but to test scenarios. And in this case, the modelling that had been leaked to the newspaper was imagining a worst-case situation, where Omicron proved very severe and thousands of Australians fell critically ill.

It was a particularly concerning time for Kelly and other public health officials. Although it was clear that caution was warranted in the face of a more infectious strain of Covid arriving during the nation's peak festive season, there was a sense that Australian authorities were rapidly running out of their social licence to ask more of the public. Perhaps they had already exhausted it. Melbourne had spent 262 days in lockdown. Sydney had been shut down for 106.

The country had been effectively cut off from the rest of the world for almost two years. Australians had been promised that if they got two doses of coronavirus vaccines, life would return to normal, or close to it. 'If we really wanted to do something, we would have had to cancel Christmas,' Kelly told us in an interview almost a year later. 'And that was not an option, partly because of a real sense of a potential for a loss of social cohesion.'

The horror scenarios of overflowing intensive-care units were avoided, but the number of infections and the severe pressures on hospitals were not. Covid cases in Australia rose exponentially over Christmas and into the summer holidays. Soon, the nation was recording more infections in a single day than it had in the entire first year and a half of the pandemic. Officially, cases peaked at 150,702 on 13 January, but by then the nation's testing system was severely overwhelmed, meaning the real number was likely to have been substantially higher. It was probably even higher than that 200,000 milestone some people had considered ridiculous.

As Christmas had approached that year, it felt like things could only be heading in one direction. After their respective lockdowns were lifted in October, many people in Victoria, New South Wales, and the Australian Capital Territory were desperately looking forward to reclaiming their freedoms. They welcomed more guests in their homes. They made bookings at restaurants. They gathered for Christmas office parties. For the first time in 582 days, a plane load of passengers from Los Angeles walked straight off their flight at Sydney Airport and into the embrace of their friends and family, as large-scale travel without quarantine resumed in November.

It was around this time that the World Health Organisation declared a new strain of Covid-19, first discovered in South Africa, 'a variant of concern', and named it Omicron. Many were keen to latch on to early reports that the variant was milder than previous iterations, even as a growing number of Australia's leading epidemiologists and public health advisers warned that, even if that was the case, the sheer number of cases could result in hospitals being overwhelmed and large-scale deaths. Australia's reopening plan had been based on the assumption that the country would still be dealing with a Delta outbreak, not the most infectious strain of Covid-19 that the world had seen.

By this point, New South Wales had a new premier. Gladys Berejiklian had sensationally resigned in October, just a few days before Sydney's lockdown had been due to be lifted, when the state's corruption watchdog had announced it was investigating whether she had breached public trust during her secret relationship with disgraced former MP Daryl Maguire. The new premier, Dominic Perrottet, wasted little time in fast-tracking the reopening. And as the new Omicron variant spread with unprecedented speed, the New South Wales government decided in mid-December to push on with a plan to drastically reduce pandemic restrictions, despite close-to-universal condemnation from public health experts.

Perrottet believed that the time for mandates was over and that the era of 'personal responsibility' had begun. 'We are treating the people of our state like adults,' he said, as daily cases of Covid in New South Wales ticked above 2,500. 'I completely accept that people are concerned. But it is our job as a government to provide confidence … There will always be new variants of this virus. The pandemic is not going away. We need to learn to live alongside it.' From 15 December, masks were no longer mandated in shops or restaurants in New South Wales. Density limits in indoor venues were also scrapped. Up to 20,000 people were allowed at music festivals.

Professor John Kaldor, an epidemiologist from the Kirby Institute, said that Australia's public health officials were very concerned that politicians were 'pretty much bent' on ending Australia's era of Covid restrictions when the severity of Omicron wasn't properly understood. 'I thought it was a big jump. We'd been having these top-down measures going on for years that [had] been aimed at protecting public health, and all of a sudden we're saying, "Oh, it's just individual responsibility,"' he said. 'I thought that leap into the unknown with this new variant was very risky.'

Kaldor, Doherty Institute head Sharon Lewin, and epidemiologist Greg Dore decided to make a rare and notable public stand
on government policy. In an opinion piece published in *The Sydney
Morning Herald* on 19 December, they called for mandatory mask
rules to be temporarily reinstated in public places and for the closure
of nightclubs for a couple of weeks. Kaldor said he showed a draft of
the article to New South Wales chief health officer Dr Kerry Chant,
who urged them to focus on pushing for measures that were most
likely to be accepted by politicians. Soon after, a letter was sent to
prime minister Scott Morrison and state and territory leaders by the
country's chief medical officer, Paul Kelly, on behalf of the Australian
Health Protection Principal Committee, with a similar message.
'Masks should be mandated in all indoor settings including retail,
hospitality when not eating or drinking, and entertainment facilities,'
Kelly wrote.

The Victorian government heeded the call just before Christmas,
beefing up its mask rules to require people aged eight or older to wear
face coverings everywhere indoors except private homes. However,
Victorian health minister Martin Foley rejected advice from the state's
chief health officer, Professor Brett Sutton, to take some further steps
to try to slow the spread of Omicron, in order to allow more time for
Victorians to receive a booster vaccination. This would have seen
dance floors closed and density caps reinstated in cafés and other
hospitality venues. The same day, as 5,715 new Covid cases were
recorded in New South Wales, and enormous queues were reported
at state testing sites, Perrottet bowed to the mounting pressure to
reinstate indoor mask mandates, bringing the state into line with
Victoria, Queensland, the ACT, and Tasmania. Morrison had earlier
argued in favour of shifting to a phase of personal responsibility in
managing Covid-19, which meant that, 'The time for that heavy hand
is behind us … We have to move from a culture of mandates to a
culture of responsibility,' he said.

Paul Kelly told us that he regretted not being stronger in his
advice during this time, in December 2021. If he had a chance to

do things again, perhaps his counsel would have been to 'slow down a bit', to give authorities a little more time to roll out the third dose of Covid vaccines. However, he also stressed that it was not his job to make decisions, but to advise those making them. 'The decisions in a democracy have to be made by our politicians, and they have to weigh up a whole bunch of other stuff that the medical experts don't have to,' Kelly said. 'Whilst I take those things into account, as I'm thinking through proportionate measures, they're the ones that have to make those decisions, and they were really hard decisions people made. What's the right decision? We'll probably never know. But the reality was the promise had been made, "If you get vaccinated, we'll get out of this." To go, "Oh, actually, it's all changed, and we need to lock down the whole country"—it would just not have worked.'

Australia's first Omicron outbreak was so large that the outbreaks that preceded it were almost wiped off the graph—they looked so small in comparison. Rather than a gradual, curved wave, it caused a close-to-vertical upwards line of cases. In the first two months of 2022, there were nearly 2.5 million cases in Australia, and likely many more not recorded, compared to fewer than 400,000 infections detected in the first two years of the pandemic. Australia would have faced a catastrophe that summer, likely on the scale seen in Italy and New York in 2020, if not for the nation's very high rate of vaccination: close to 94 per cent of Australians aged over 16 years had by this point received at least two doses. Critically, Australians also took matters into their own hands in the absence of strict Covid rules, voluntarily restricting their movements and socialising to a point that resembled a lockdown in some places. In the first week of January 2022, for example, Victorians reduced their movements to levels very close to what was seen during the strict 'stage four' lockdown the year before.

'It flattened the curve [of cases],' explained leading pandemic adviser Professor James McCaw. 'Our hospital system was under extreme pressure, but it didn't collapse. But it would have if we had not changed our behaviour … It's a success of the community and a success for public health messaging as well.'

The first Omicron wave caused Australia's testing system to temporarily collapse, hospitals were pushed close to the edge of their capacity—and sometimes beyond it—and an unprecedented number of Australians died of Covid. One paramedic service was so understaffed that surf lifesavers, students, and other volunteers were brought in to drive ambulances. Surgeons in Sydney were emailed asking for their help in filling basic ward shifts, and were told that their hospital was facing a 'crisis of epic proportions'. In an extraordinary step usually reserved for bushfires and mass-casualty events, a 'code brown' was declared for Victoria's major hospitals, with many operations cancelled in a bid to ration limited beds and staff. The state's triple-zero system was also overwhelmed by the extra demand, and dozens of people died after calls for an ambulance were left waiting. Boxes of Covid swabs piled up at pathology testing clinics, untouched, amid a tsunami of demand for testing. It was so difficult to find rapid home-testing kits at pharmacies, nicknamed RATs, that people were reselling them online for up to ten times their retail price.

The Morrison government was blamed for the RAT debacle. They had been warned for months that they should secure more of the testing kits. Britain, famously, had ample free test kits available for the community. In the end, state governments were forced to take the very measures the experts had advised many weeks earlier. Both Victoria and New South Wales banned indoor dance floors in January as Covid hospitalisations piled up. *The Sydney Morning Herald* described the move in New South Wales as 'a major reversal of Premier Dominic Perrottet's insistence that New South Wales would stay open despite the high caseload'.

The adjustment to living with Covid-19 was a particular shock for states that for most of the pandemic had only experienced a handful of cases. When Tasmania lifted its border restrictions in mid-December with 90 per cent of its eligible population vaccinated, the island state went from having virtually no cases over 20 months to many hundreds of cases a day by January. The state government, like the government of South Australia, was criticised by some for not delaying its reopening until at least after Christmas. The Tasmanian premier Peter Gutwein decided to push ahead because of advice that the warmer summer months would be the best time to deal with the disease. 'If we waited, it would have meant we were then dealing with this as the seasons were then starting to turn, and it would have been more problematic,' he said.

Tasmanians had become accustomed to the idea of people with Covid-19 being outsiders. The state's top public health official, Dr Mark Veitch, said now they had to explain to Tasmanians that 'the people with Covid would be us'. Within a few weeks, authorities stopped listing individual sites that had been visited by confirmed Covid cases, as had been the practice for so long. Dr Veitch said this was because the whole state of Tasmania was basically an exposure site. It was the same situation everywhere, except for Western Australia.

CHAPTER TWENTY

Western Australia, the 'island within an island'

It is impossible to separate Western Australia's unique experience of coronavirus from its premier, Mark McGowan, who emerged from the pandemic the world's most popular political leader. Invisible borders defined the pandemic nationally, but perhaps no more so than in isolated Western Australia, where the state was shut off to much of the country and the world for 697 days. McGowan's hardline policies often stoked fierce controversy elsewhere, but resulted in a cult-like, rockstar fandom at home, where his approval rating skyrocketed to almost 90 per cent. Young children knew his name. Diehard fans tattooed his face onto their bodies. One tattoo, on a man's leg, immortalised the 55-year-old premier's face wearing a bandana and making a 'W' sign with his fingers above the words 'Westside bitches'. When shown the picture at a press conference, McGowan offered suggestions for laser tattoo removal. An image of his head adorned cereal boxes in a limited-edition line called 'State Daddy O's.' His appeal only grew after he made national headlines making light about a man who stopped to eat a kebab when running from police, coining the phrase: 'There's nothing unlawful about going for a run and eating a kebab.'

In early April 2020, as the Ruby Princess outbreak was unravelling in New South Wales, and Australia had just recorded its 24th death from coronavirus, McGowan did something that would supercharge his remarkable popularity: he announced a hard border banning all travel into Western Australia, with limited exemptions, to pursue Covid-zero. 'These new harder border closures essentially mean we will be turning Western Australia into its own island, within an island—our own country,' McGowan declared. A state of disaster had been announced in Western Australia on 16 March 2020, giving the government the ability to close the borders at will, a feature that defined McGowan's leadership.

'Isolation—it was our biggest advantage,' McGowan said bluntly, speaking from his minimalist reddish, brown-timber office at Parliament House in Perth in the early spring of 2022. A small group of protestors were chanting on the steps outside in the sun, demanding an end to greyhound racing. 'It might get in somewhere else, but we could stop it because we can isolate ourselves from the rest of Australia.'

McGowan gained a national reputation for snapping his state's borders shut as soon as a single case emerged in Victoria and New South Wales—or any other state, for that matter. By mid-April 2020, the state's hardline approach had eliminated the community transmission of coronavirus, becoming one of the few places in the world to do so. Remote learning for schools was in place for only a few weeks in March and April 2020, and the economy boomed. West Australians spent just 12 days in three separate lockdowns in 2021. When McGowan lifted the restrictions on pub service following Australia's first national shutdown in 2020, a tavern in his electorate of Rockingham, the Swinging Pig, celebrated by offering free meals to everyone named Mark, Marc, Marcus, or Marco, and promised to shout the whole pub a pint if the premier turned up. During a press conference, McGowan vowed to visit the tavern, and stayed true to his word. The pub was full of Marks, and McGowan arrived to a rockstar welcome.

Between mid-April 2020 and the end of 2021, only a handful of coronavirus cases of community transmission would be reported in the state, which is roughly the size of western Europe and has a population of more than 2.6 million. But in late December 2021, an unvaccinated but infected French backpacker arrived, starting a cluster that would infect more than 20 people and spark the closures of nightclubs, the cancellation of music festivals, and a temporary mandatory mask rule in all indoor settings and on public transport.

McGowan had planned on flying back to the eastern states the week after the meeting on 13 March 2020 of state leaders and prime minister Morrison in Parramatta. Instead, he would not fly to Australia's eastern states for more than two years. He cleared his diary, and met with the state disaster council, led by former West Australian police commissioner Chris Dawson. As the top unelected official in managing the pandemic, Dawson had the power to sign directions restricting movements within and into the state, as well as other measures that would usually have to be passed through parliament. In the early months, McGowan, a former naval officer, spent hours each day with his team, including health minister Roger Cook and the chief health officer, Dr Andy Robertson, wargaming how the state would respond.

'Every day, the situation was getting bigger and bigger. All the news from around the world just grew like an avalanche,' McGowan said, spinning his hands to mimic a snowball rolling down a hill. The speed at which the pandemic unfolded left McGowan struggling to process the magnitude of it all the time. 'I was just shocked,' he said. 'I kept thinking: is this *really* happening? Are we *really* going to do this?' Robertson was staying up late at night, reading everything he could about the virus so he could brief Cook and McGowan. 'There was considerable trepidation at that time,' Robertson said. 'We didn't know how effective any of the measures like social distancing would even be.'

If there was ever a moment when the pandemic truly arrived in Western Australia, most people at the heart of the coronavirus response there will tell you it was when the coronavirus-plagued

Artania cruise ship quietly docked south of Perth. The German vessel, with more than 800 people on board, was only meant to refuel before disembarking. But an outbreak onboard would eventually result in four passengers dying and dozens more falling seriously ill, triggering a political storm that spiralled into a tense stand-off between Western Australia and the federal government.

McGowan described the fiasco as one of the greatest frustrations of his life, and said he was terrified the cruise ship would somehow let the virus into the state and quickly overrun hospitals. 'The most dramatic thing up front was stopping the cruise ships,' he said. 'The police commissioner was showing us every morning on his app the cruise ships coming across from Melbourne or Sydney. We were worried they were all going to come into Fremantle … we were sending messages, "You can't come in, you've got to go home."'

McGowan had just seen off the Swiss-owned Magnifica cruise—not without its own drama. Days earlier, the Magnifica had sailed through Perth, stopping once in Fremantle to refuel, with no passengers disembarking, before it continued on to Dubai McGowan had issued a stern warning that unless it was a medical emergency, nobody would be getting off. 'I will not allow what happened in Sydney to happen here.'

Days later, when the Artania sailed towards Perth, McGowan vowed that no one on board the ship—passengers mostly from Germany, Austria, and Switzerland—would set foot on dry land, leaving the vessel stranded for days. He was adamant that the 230-metre–long ship, which was on a 140-night around-the-world cruise, with nine decks, 832 passengers, and 503 crew, was a Commonwealth responsibility, and demanded they take charge of the crew and passengers. 'The federal government needs to step up here,' a visibly frustrated McGowan told reporters on 25 March 2020, when the ship emerged on Perth's shores. 'Get the ship away, and get them home.'

It was during the Artania debacle that West Australia's health minister, Roger Cook, and the federal health minister, Greg Hunt, both called Perth anaesthetist Andrew Miller on the same day. 'They were very upset with me, and they made that very clear to me,' said Miller, the-then head of the Western Australian branch of the Australian Medical Association, with a hint of amusement in his voice. The catalyst for these calls was a move by the doctors' lobby group, led by Miller, to push back against a state govern- ment plan to admit dozens of passengers and crew from the ship to the three private hospitals in Perth: the Bethesda, the Mount, and Hollywood.

Miller, who worked at the hospitals, sensed a potential disaster. 'We stepped over a line, and said that we would support doctors with- drawing service from those hospitals,' Miller said. 'It was probably the most risky call that I've made through this whole pandemic. But it was an open ICU at Hollywood and at the Mount hospitals, with no prospect of isolating people from airborne spread. I knew that none of them were prepared for this. People who were being called in that weekend had not been through Covid training.'

Hunt called Miller after the doctor's objection to the plan was reported in the media. Miller said he was sitting on the edge of his bed experiencing the full force of a 'Greg Hunt missile'. Miller said Hunt asked him if he wanted to become famous for being the doctor around the world who was refusing to treat coronavirus patients.

'And I said, "Well, that's just not the case. We just don't want them to be treated in an inappropriate facility. In many cases, it will be the same doctors, in fact, who will be treating them. They just want the tools to do their job properly."' Miller suggested to Hunt that the sick passengers be sent to the Joondalup Health Campus, a 145-bed private hospital in the northern suburbs of Perth, which had negative-pressure isolation rooms for patients with infectious diseases.

'By the end of that phone call, things had really turned around, and [Hunt] said, "Well, you're someone I can work with, and we can get this done,"' Miller recalled. Miller's correspondence with Hunt remained sporadically effective, but was tense after the Artania episode.

Hunt recalled being horrified when Western Australia refused to land the Artania ship, and contacted a Liberal Senate member for Western Australia, Mathias Cormann. 'Mathias and I thought it was just an outrage,' Hunt said. 'We could see a shipload of people who could all catch it, of which there could be hundreds of deaths, so we worked with Roger Cook, who was fantastic. He was doing everything he could to get it landed, and it was being resisted by senior members of the government.' Hunt said the agreement to have the Joondalup Hospital take patients came about because the chief executive of the health service was close friends with Cormann, and told the senator he was confident the hospital was ready to handle Covid cases.

West Australian orthopaedic surgeon and former national president of the influential Australian Medical Association, Omar Khorshid, has mostly praised the way the Western Australian government handled the early years of the pandemic. But he said that of all the dramatic events that unfolded in Australia during the pandemic, his hometown's initial reaction to the Artania sits most uncomfortably with him. 'I was very disappointed with Mark McGowan at the time,' Khorshid said. 'I thought his behaviour was despicable, to be frank. We had this ship, which was said to be full of very, very sick Germans. There was the potential that people were going to die on the ship that had come towards WA for help.' Khorshid said a disaster was averted in the case of the Artania by backroom politics; but, years later, he cannot shake the feeling that there was an element of xenophobia to it all. 'Do you want Australia to be seen as a country that doesn't help out?' he said. 'It is not part of our identity. So I found that very challenging.'

A passenger's medical emergency, which was unrelated to coronavirus, meant that the Antarnia did eventually have to dock in Perth. It led to prime minister Scott Morrison intervening, arguing that Australia had a moral and humanitarian obligation to care for the Covid-infected passengers onboard. At the same time, the Vasco da Gama cruise ship was also floating precariously close to Perth, and Morrison ordered the state to quarantine the 800 passengers in limbo. They were shipped off to Rottnest Island for 14 days of quarantine in hotels.

McGowan lost sleep over trying to deal with three cruise ships arriving at the Fremantle port within the one week, all demanding help to deal with ill or Covid-infected passengers. There were only 160 intensive-care beds in the entire state at the time. More than 40 people were taken to hospital from the Artania. After a saga that included 24 days being docked in Fremantle, 81 positive Covid-19 cases, a series of mercy flights from Australia to Germany, the deaths of four people—including three passengers and a crew member—a wedding on board, and a spate of peculiar claims by passengers, including that a sick doctor had been going 'from cabin to cabin, absolutely unprotected', the ill-fated ship finally left Western Australia.

The brokered arrangement with the state and federal governments about what to do with the Atarnia, led by doctors, including Miller, set the scene for the months that followed. In Western Australia, Miller was often a lone voice calling for quicker, stronger action from the state and federal governments over the airborne spread of Covid-19. He hit a sweet spot with many in the west, who believed he was talking sense and keeping them safe.

Miller said he was in a relentless pursuit to protect Australian healthcare workers from the fate of places such as Italy, where doctors and nurses were dying in their dozens. He would often criticise the government or goad them in the media, pushing for more protective gear for healthcare workers or for more Covid testing clinics. For a while, whatever he was pushing for was rejected, before being announced soon afterwards by Cook or McGowan. Miller noted that his relationship with former chief medical officer Brendan Murphy also became strained after Miller publicly criticised him for being too slow to grasp many aspects of the pandemic, including the importance of masks.

'It's not my job to get along with people,' Miller told us from his home in Perth. 'My job is to represent the views of doctors and other healthcare workers who don't have a voice. What I do understand is the duplicity of governments and health services. It was very clear to me that these organisations don't tell the truth or pursue science—that's not their modus operandi. Everything is through a political lens and through a budgetary lens.'

A constant fear of Miller's was that the virus would get into Western Australia's Indigenous communities, and wreak devastation there. In Broome, a town in the Kimberley region where roughly one-third of the population is Aboriginal, Miller led a public push to improve infection control at the local hospital, concerned that a coronavirus outbreak there could mean gravely ill patients would die by the time it took them to fly to Perth. The hospital now has among the best infection-protection controls in Australia.

Miller said most politicians avoided him like the plague after the pandemic was declared, but he did have one fleeting and comical interaction with McGowan during an episode of the current affairs show *Flashpoint* at the start of the pandemic. Miller, concerned about shaking people's hands due to coronavirus, inadvertently offended McGowan after the premier stuck out his hand to the doctor before the two appeared on television together. 'I didn't shake his hand, and I think he thought I was snobbing him,' Miller said. 'It was before everyone had gotten into the don't-shake-hands part of the pandemic.' Before Miller could explain, McGowan was whisked off by his minders.

The closed borders in Western Australia were a sore point in Canberra, and as result, McGowan's relationship with Morrison was strained at times. In late August 2021, McGowan publicly rejected Morrison's national reopening plan, declaring he would not 'deliberately import the virus' by throwing open the borders to New South Wales, where thousands of infections were being reported every week. Morrison used a television appearance on the *Today* show to compare the border debate to a fictional cartoon about a prehistoric family. 'Now, it's like that movie—in *The Croods*, people wanted to stay in the cave ... and that young girl, she wanted to go out and live again, and deal with the challenges of living in a different world,' Morrison told host Karl Stefanovic.

McGowan interpreted this as a slight, comparing West Australians to cave people. 'I think everyone would rather just see the Commonwealth look beyond New South Wales and actually appreciate what life is like here in WA,' McGowan retaliated on Facebook. 'We currently have no restrictions within our state, a great quality of life, and a remarkably strong economy which is funding the relief efforts in other parts of the country … West Aussies just want decisions that consider the circumstances of all States and Territories, not just Sydney.'

The two clashed publicly on several more occasions, including when McGowan accused Morrison of dog-whistling to 'anti-vaccination terrorists' after the prime minister spoke out against broad vaccine mandates, saying he sympathised with the frustrations of Australians. Morrison's comments came days after Western Australia had mandated immunisations to tackle a lagging uptake. This was a particularly stressful time for McGowan, who received a barrage of death threats over the mandates after his phone number was leaked online. He remembered stepping out of an event at a local RSL to find about 50 text messages and dozens of missed calls on this phone. 'It was like, "You effing grub, we're gonna kill you,"' McGowan recalled. 'They were threatening to kill my children. We ended up having the police at the house for six months around the clock. Some of them [the callers] were so dumb, they called on their own mobile numbers and left death threats.'

But despite their disagreements over matters such as vaccine mandates, in the more than 60 national cabinet meetings they took part in, McGowan said Morrison was always meticulous and across his brief. Behind the scenes, they were affable, there was mutual respect, and they spoke on the phone regularly, although their conversations often quickly descended into heated debates or arguments. The premier would push back against Morrison, who was adamant that Western Australia follow the national plan for reopening when the state reached an 80 per cent vaccinated rate. 'We'd have these arguments—it was like Groundhog Day all the time,' McGowan said.

McGowan's popularity only soared further when he took on billionaire mining giant and former politician Clive Palmer, who publicly opposed the Western Australia border closures. For the most part of 2021, Palmer and McGowan were locked in a bitter dispute about the premier's decision to close the state's borders. The Queensland mining magnate claimed he was brought into 'hatred, ridicule and contempt' after Mr McGowan called him an 'enemy of the state' over his High Court challenge seeking to overturn Western Australia's hard border policy.

Seared in McGowan's memory is the former prime minister calling him while Morrison was cooking a curry for his family one night, urging him to drop the Palmer case. 'He rang me, and he said our legal advice is you're going to get done, you're going to lose,' McGowan recalled with amusement. 'I said our legal advice is the opposite, that we are going to win. He said, no you're wrong, the Commonwealth solicitor-general's told us you're going to lose, so don't go through the embarrassment, Mark, trust me, don't go through the embarrassment.' McGowan stood firm: 'I told him I'm not doing it, just so you know, I am not giving in on the borders to Clive Palmer. I will not. That's it. Thank you. You can keep talking about it to me, but I'm not doing it.'

McGowan said he did not dislike Morrison, like other people in the national cabinet seemed to. 'In fact, I liked him. With those two exceptions, he was always reasonable and friendly to me. I didn't have this hostility that I've heard from other premiers.'

When we asked Morrison about which states he thought had the best pandemic response, he first replied that South Australia had done an exceptional job in getting the balance right. Of the Covid-zero states, South Australia had been the quickest to reopen its domestic borders in 2021, in line with the national plan. Then he added that, as much as he did not like domestic border closures, when it came to Western Australia, already so physically isolated, he understood it. In 2023, Western Australia had achieved the lowest rate of death from Covid in Australia, alongside the Australian Capital Territory and the Northern Territory.

'There's a lot said about the arguments that I had about domestic borders. Well, to be honest, I learnt,' Morrison said. 'As much as I didn't like domestic borders, in the case of Western Australia, I could see how it made sense … you can have differences of view about when they came off and how they are exercised, and all the rest of it, but the actual use of them, I think it's hard to argue against, certainly not.' However, Morrison argued that the closure of Western Australia's border, which runs through hundreds of kilometres of desert in some of the remotest parts of the country, had very different impacts from the closures that divided populated and tightly knit communities in New South Wales and Queensland, and had much more far-reaching consequences, such as preventing people from getting urgent medical care.

'I'm not necessarily criticising [Queensland premier Annastacia Palaszczuk], that was her call, but … the borders impacted differently in diffferent places because of the geography,' Morrison said.

When quizzed about his relationship with the other state leaders, McGowan said he always found New South Wales premier Gladys Berejiklian 'to be very difficult'. McGowan's view was that New South Wales was 'always arrogant' without just cause. 'They were always the gold standard, but then they'd have these huge issues, and then spread it to us,' McGowan said. 'That was always very difficult, because the New South Wales government wouldn't do what was required. They were a bit of a basket case. Victoria had it, but they were never triumphalist like New South Wales was.'

In one of his many public jabs at New South Wales, McGowan announced on Facebook in March 2021 that he had put in a paper shredder a bill for more than $7 million that the New South Wales government had sent his state for quarantining returned travellers in hotels. Months later, he threw another $5 million hotel quarantine bill from New South Wales premier Dominic Perrottet in the bin. Yet McGowan expressed deep respect for other state leaders that he worked alongside in the pandemic. He considers South Australia's former premier Steven Marshall and Queensland premier

Annastacia Palaszczuk as friends, and told us that former Northern Territory chief minister Michael Gunner 'was everyone's favourite on the national cabinet'.

McGowan also said he had never encountered a politician to be more across the facts, including the nitty-gritty details, than Daniel Andrews. 'He's got a very, very sharp intellect.' At the height of Victoria's outbreaks, McGowan said he texted Andrews several messages of support: 'Can we help? What can we do?' He remembered feeling strange calling him, concerned that he might come across as insensitive or boasting, adding that he struggled to empathise with Andrews and the grim situation he faced. 'I couldn't offer him any advice, because what do I say?' he said. 'He says, "Oh, we've had 5,000 cases. Twenty people have died. Our hospitals are overrun." And I say, "We've got no cases, and our economy is going ahead." How do I empathise? Because it was such a different story here.'

McGowan said no other premier in Australia wanted to be Andrews during the consecutive lockdowns and outbreaks of 2020. 'We, Queensland, the Northern Territory, South Australia, and Tasmania would always be looking at what was going on there, thinking, *But for the grace of God … My God, I don't want to be in that position*,' McGowan said. 'We all felt for Dan. I was always watching Victoria, thinking, *I don't want to get there*.' For months, McGowan switched on the evening news to watch the crisis gripping Melbourne as journalists relayed the Victorian news of the day. McGowan said this only strengthened his resolve about his own hard border closures. 'Suburbs, the whole city locked down, people were dying. People were locked in public housing blocks. It was awful. And it was like, well, what are my choices?' he said.

McGowan's strong stance on border closures stirred up memories for many of the long streak of separatist feelings that has defined Western Australia throughout its history, frequently placing it at odds with its eastern neighbours. Western Australia is the only state to have tried to secede from the Australian federation, a move attempted in the 1930s. There are also striking parallels between the Spanish Flu pandemic and the Covid pandemic 100 years later; most notably in McGown's steadfast approach echoing that of another Western Australian premier, Hal Colebatch. In 1919, during the Spanish Flu pandemic, there was bickering between the state and the Commonwealth when Colebatch temporarily halted the new transcontinental train service from Melbourne. Passengers were set up in tents and marquees near Kalgoorlie, but the wind blew down the tents, and the train's dining and sleeping cars had to be used instead. 'Spanish influenza did eventually penetrate WA's borders,' wrote Carolyn Holbrook, a historian at Deakin University in Melbourne. 'But the delay in onset probably diluted its virulence. Of the 12,000 Australians who died from Spanish influenza, less than 650 were West Australians.'

The Australian National University's Professor Mark Kenny theorised in an interview with *The Age* in 2022 that McGowan's popularity was partly a result of circumstance, but also of his deep and rich understanding of West Australians and his ability to communicate that clearly. 'Plain speaking is one of McGowan's great strengths … he speaks very clearly and persuasively and in normal language—there's a lot of purpose behind his communications,' Kenny said. 'What makes him successful is that he understands very clearly that it is West Australians that he answers to, and no one else.' McGowan's popularity in the west during the pandemic saw him secure a landslide election victory in March 2021. His party obliterated the Liberals, reducing them to two seats.

The long-awaited reopening of Western Australia came on 3 March 2022, after the hottest summer on record, a flood-induced food-supply crisis, and a sweeping Omicron outbreak pushed daily infections in the country's eastern states into the thousands. The initially announced plan had been to reopen the border almost a month earlier, on 5 February 2022, but McGowan found himself reconsidering that decision while holidaying with his family on Rottnest Island. During this trip, McGowan told us he was constantly fielding calls, texts, and emails from elderly people and local business owners, urging him to stall the reopening. He came around to that view, and in an evening press conference held on 20 January, he announced the delayed reopening, blaming escalating health risks and low third-dose vaccination rates. He said previous plans to reopen had been based on the less transmissible Delta variant, arguing that the 'world changed when Omicron arrived' and that it would be reckless to reopen.

The distress of not seeing his own family members, who had already booked flights to come to Perth from overseas, got the better of the typically level-headed Omar Khorshid. The orthopaedic surgeon sent off a series of late-night tweets bemoaning the decision, writing that he was 'gutted', and calling McGown a 'one-trick pony'. He argued that the state needed to prepare for Omicron as it was already in Australia, and that 'sticking our head in the sand won't make it go away'. He went to bed and fell asleep. But at 2.00 am his phone started ringing. He switched it on silent, and went back to sleep. When he woke up, there were 27 missed calls from a producer at the *Today* show, and at least 50 further separate media requests. 'They really wanted me on, but I didn't want to add fuel to the little fire that I'd started,' Khorshid said. More than a year later, Khorshid's view remained that the borders could have opened on 5 February as planned. 'Nothing was going to stop Omicron,' he said.

The decision to delay reopening would give McGowan the political fright of his career. His approval rating plummeted to about 63 per cent almost overnight. During that extra month, however, third-dose vaccination rates jumped from 25 per cent to 70 per cent. 'I know there was a lot of carry-on, but it was only a month,' McGowan said. 'We will never know how many, but a whole bunch of people are alive who may have otherwise been dead.'

Most Western Australians would say that the state had the best experience during Covid, Khorshid said, but there was a price to pay. 'You'll find 80 per cent of people very happy with the response, and about 20 per cent were quite unhappy because of borders,' he said. 'Families suffered, people weren't able to get to funerals and weddings. There was definitely a cost, but almost everyone in Western Australia would agree that the cost was worth paying.'

Asked about the toll of the more than 690 days of closed borders, McGowan was quick to defend the state's hardline approach to keeping the virus out, and said that, even with the benefit of hindsight, he would do it all over again. His response to the question hinted at an underlying exasperation, and it was the only point during our extended interview with him that he appeared visibly frustrated. He emphasised that while Western Australia's borders closed on 5 April 2020 and did not fully open until 3 March 2022, the state was open to parts of Australia at various times, when there were no outbreaks of the disease spreading.

'This idea that we were closed off for two years ... it's rubbish,' he said. 'In fact, we were open to the entirety of Australia for various points in time. We were open to Queensland, Tasmania, South Australia, and the Northern Territory most of the time. Everyone says, "I couldn't come here, I couldn't go to WA ... to see my parents." We were open to New South Wales and Victoria when they didn't have Covid. It [the border] was opened and closed at times. People chose not to come during those periods.'

However, the fact remains that many people from the most populous states in the country did not see their families in Western Australia for almost two years because the 14-day mandatory quarantine and stringent travel exemptions proved insurmountable for them. Some Australians who lived outside the state did not get to say goodbye to loved ones who died, or to attend their funerals. McGowan said he has always had compassion for people separated by the pandemic from those they loved. He noted that he did not see his own elderly parents, both in their 80s, who live in rural New South Wales, where he grew up, for more than a year.

'But as the premier of the state, you have an obligation to protect people,' McGowan said. 'I was watching the news every night, like everyone, and there were these mass graves in New York and Italy. People [were] dying on the street in China. In Britain, thousands of people [were] dying every day. I had to do everything here to stop this thing,' McGowan said. 'I felt strongly that I had to do what needed to be done.'

By the end of 2022, Western Australia had had the lowest coronavirus death rates in the nation during the Omicron wave. An official analysis of registered Covid-19 deaths undertaken by the Australia Bureau of Statistics, when standardised for different age groups, showed that Western Australia, which had shut out the rest of Australia and the world for an extended period, has been the most successful jurisdiction in limiting Covid-19 deaths. Western Australia reported 15 deaths per 100,000 people during the Omicron wave, compared to New South Wales' 33.4 and Victoria's 33.1. Western Australia lived in almost serene normality compared to Victoria's gruelling coronavirus outbreaks and lockdowns of 2020 and 2021, and yet some of the country's most bizarre quarantine breaches occurred in the isolated state.

Andy Robertson, the chief health officer, still remains unsure why Western Australia was able to avoid some of the super-spreading events that New South Wales and Victoria fell victim to, but suspects the hard borders helped, along with a bit of good luck. 'People here weren't behaving like monks — they were attending events and going to the gym,' he said. 'We had some cases pop up, but, for whatever reason, they were fortunately poor spreaders.'

The cases came from all over the country. At the Great Eastern Motor Lodge in Rivervale, an inner-eastern suburb of Perth, Brisbane man Travis Myles, who was in the midst of a 14-day quarantine, escaped his fourth-storey room by climbing out of his window and down a makeshift bedsheet rope. A South Australian father-of-four, Glen Tonkin, was sentenced to two months' imprisonment after leaving self-quarantine on day 12 and visiting the Northbridge Brewing Company in Perth for a drink. (He never spent time in custody after a successful appeal against the sentence.) And a 20-year-old Perth aviation student also successfully appealed his two-month sentence for sneaking out of isolation to visit a woman on day 13 of his self-quarantine.

But the most staggering breach was by Melbourne bar and restaurant owner Hayden Burbank and financial planner Mark Babbage, who were arrested, charged, and jailed for three months after having entered Western Australia by falsely claiming to be Northern Territory residents so they could attend the AFL grand final to watch the Melbourne Demons play against the Western Bulldogs. They went to the trouble of falsifying a Northern Territory driver's licence to support their applications. Their plan came undone in spectacular fashion when a photo on the AFL's Instagram account showed Burbank and Babbage alongside Melbourne player Alex Neal-Bullen inside the Demons' locker rooms, celebrating and drinking with players after the club's 57-year-drought-breaking win. For a second year in a row, the 2021 AFL Grand Final was held away from its traditional home of the Melbourne Cricket Ground as, again in lockdown, the city watched one of its teams secure victory in another state. It was the first grand final to be held in Perth, and it set a new record for AFL attendance in Western Australia. More than 61,000 spectators filled the city's Optus Stadium to the rafters.

In May 2023, McGowan called time on his nearly three-decade career in politics, including six years as premier, citing 'burnout,' a type of mental, physical, and emotional exhaustion typically sparked by being relentlessly overworked. It came almost six months after former New Zealand prime minister Jacinda Ardern resigned, also citing burnout in the aftermath of the pandemic. McGowan said that, for him, burnout had manifested as 'sleepless nights' and 'excess worry about things'. He described the role as premier as 'all-consuming' and revealed he no longer had the drive to continue.

'But the truth is, I am tired. Extremely tired. In fact, I'm exhausted … Now is the right time to step aside from the job I love,' McGowan told reporters at a press conference on 29 May 2022, flanked by his wife, Sarah. 'The Covid experience, basically three years standing here … and all the pressures associated with that, that drained me a lot. I'm pretty much spent now, so I will hand over to someone else.'

When McGowan was asked what stories he would be telling

about the pandemic in years to come, his eyes lit up as he recounted a story about his daughter Amelia. It was in the frantic hours before a lockdown, and he and Amelia were at the Coles supermarket in the beachside suburb of Rockingham, rushing to stock up on supplies. She was weaving and ducking through crowds, grabbing bundles of toilet paper for a group of elderly ladies who were anxiously waiting outside the supermarket. The women were afraid of venturing into the chaotic scene as hundreds of people panic-shopped, elbowing each other out of the way, stripping the shelves of food and toilet paper.

'She was running a gauntlet to get the toilet paper out to the old ladies,' McGowan recalled, chuckling at the memory. The image of his daughter running through Coles in the hours before lockdown is a scenario most Australians who lived through the pandemic can relate to, and it is one of McGowan's most enduring memories of that time. 'The toilet paper wars. That was all so weird,' he said.

CHAPTER TWENTY-ONE

Living with Covid

Sherene Magana Cruz's voice cracked as she spoke. 'You've got me on a really emotional day,' she said. 'I feel like the world is moving on, but I'm not.' It was 2023, and the 51-year-old was still living with the crippling, lingering symptoms of a Covid infection she had caught while working at a Melbourne aged-care home a few years earlier. Every day, the mother of three was waking to searing pain through her shoulders, feet, hips, and ankles. She would forget simple words, lost in a daze. Standing for more than 20 minutes was excruciating. Cruz had not been able to return to her job as an aged-care worker. 'I have to keep trying to convince my doctors that, "Hey this is not normal." You can feel like you're going crazy,' she said. 'I used to be this out-there, bubbly, happy person who loved working with elderly people and supporting them, but I feel like I've just lost myself.'

As Australians began living alongside rampant Covid from the end of 2021, many people returned to busy, vibrant lives, unencumbered by rules and restrictions. However, millions of Australians were infected with the disease for the first time, and deaths soared to record levels. By 2023, it was thought that tens of thousands of Australians, like Cruz, were living with a severe form of long Covid, a condition often marked by bone-deep exhaustion, brain fog, and other life-altering symptoms. The doctors trying to support these patients, despite inadequate funding and with no proven treatment available, said they were inundated. Some had waiting lists almost a year long.

The harm wrought by Covid became even more concentrated within certain groups, who were mostly vaccinated but had other vulnerabilities. Older Australians with medical conditions were dying in their thousands. But pandemic fatigue had also set in, and people would declare that they were 'done'—done with masks, done with vaccines, and done with Covid, even if it wasn't done with them. Almost all government-imposed restrictions in Australia were lifted by the spring of 2022. While most agreed that the time for sweeping rules was over, governments stopped talking so much about how people should navigate the risks they still faced. Victoria's chief health officer, Brett Sutton, who had appeared at press conferences almost daily for a couple of years, was not made available for a media conference for more than 10 months until the day his resignation was announced in June 2023.

Infectious disease physician Dr Paul Griffin described this as a strategy of extremes. 'It was a little too harsh early on, when the risk perception was perhaps too high and our response lacked nuance,' he said. 'Then we became, seemingly almost overnight, very liberal and relaxed. Now it's really challenging to actually try and get support for any measures to address Covid and the real risk it still poses in the community.'

Mark Butler, who became Australia's federal health minister in 2022, told us there was a group of people that was still quite exercised and frightened by Covid-19, 'but the broad bulk of the population don't want to talk about it, and want to move on'. This put authorities in a difficult position. Governments wanted to keep some goodwill in the tank, just in case they needed to ask more of Australians again. 'If a nasty new variant that causes more severe disease comes our way this year [in 2023], God forbid, then we have the headroom to escalate,' Butler said.

Talk of the pandemic was, for the most part, conspicuously absent from the federal election campaign in the autumn of 2022, even when opposition leader Anthony Albanese caught Covid in the first weeks. James Massola, *The Age* newspaper's national affairs editor, explained that internal political party and media polling was showing that voters were 'sick of it, they just wanted the pandemic to be over'. Whether voters were swayed by prime minister Scott Morrison's record of managing Covid-19 was a different question entirely.

Morrison had begun the pandemic with his reputation singed by an ill-timed family holiday to Hawaii in December 2019, where he was photographed at a beachside bar as bushfires crackled and roared across his home state. The misstep was made unforgettable by a comment he made to Sydney's 2GB radio station while still in Honolulu, preparing to return home early in the face of the public backlash. 'You know, I don't hold a hose, mate, and I don't sit in a control room,' he'd said. Casually deflecting responsibility in the face of a humanitarian and environmental crisis fuelled an emerging narrative that Morrison avoided accountability.

The advent of the biggest health and economic crisis to hit the country in the 21st century offered him an opportunity to reset, and at first it did exactly that. Morrison's approval ratings climbed through March, April, and May 2020. Voters of all stripes were grateful for the federal government's pandemic leadership, as Australia was held up for its early success in containing the disease. However, there were several things that happened later which guaranteed that the public wouldn't forget that their prime minister didn't 'hold a hose'. As most Australians clamoured for the vaccine, Morrison famously declared that the nation's vaccine rollout was 'not a race'. The following summer of 2021–2022, the federal government bore the blame for not having ordered enough rapid tests during another chaotic holiday period that was meant to have been better than the previous one.

Massola, who followed Morrison on parts of the election campaign trail, said there was also a perception among voters that the prime minister had treated the states run by Labor governments—particularly Victoria, but also Queensland and Western Australia—unfairly compared to the Liberal states. 'He'd extol New South Wales as the "gold standard" while he and his ministers, such as health minister Greg Hunt and treasurer Josh Frydenberg, would berate Victoria,' Massola said. 'I think that had a massively deleterious effect on the Coalition's vote in Victoria, but I also think it played out everywhere. I think people saw the double standard.' Massola said there was a sense among voters of a government that had run out of ideas, and was out of touch.

Albanese's Labor Party went on to secure majority government, while a high-profile group of independent women candidates running on a platform of climate change action and government integrity won a string of seats from sitting 'moderate' Liberals in affluent areas of the country. Those stripped of their seats included federal treasurer Josh Frydenberg, a Victorian who had been widely touted as a future prime minister and had also been a vigorous critic of the Victorian government's response to the pandemic. Victorian premier Daniel Andrews won a landslide third election victory in the state's November 2022 election, surprising pollsters and the political parties, who had expected a bigger lockdown backlash from voters. Labor did lose ground in its traditional working-class heartland in the north and west—the areas hardest hit by Covid-19 and pandemic restrictions. But the same impact wasn't seen in the more marginal seats, in affluent areas where people had kept their jobs during the lockdowns and were able to work from home.

Scott Morrison, the former prime minister, looked tanned and relaxed as he popped onto the video call with us, beaming in from his office in the Sutherland Shire, south of Sydney, a locale of bronze-white beaches. His grey shirt was pulled up casually to his forearms. The man who was once the most powerful person in the land had spent the last few months on the backbench of parliament, but the demotion had its perks. It was a Monday afternoon in late January 2023, and it was the MP's first day back at work after the Christmas holidays. 'The shire is always fantastic in summer,' he said, as he sipped from a black mug with the Liberal Party logo on it.

This was not the besuited politician most Australians had come to know. The refreshed holiday version of Morrison seemed keener to shore up friends than to inflame pandemic tensions. Indeed, if he was bitter or angry about the past, he did a good job of concealing it. The federal election disaster? He didn't harbour any ill-feelings about that, he said. 'I mean, it was an extraordinary period of time in the life of Australians, and there are many things that went into the election, but no doubt people wanted to put that time behind them, for better or for worse. And I think there was a sense of drawing the line. We've seen that in many countries around the world.'

Of the many politicians interviewed for this book, only a few admitted to having had a crisis of confidence as they made previously unthinkable decisions, locking down millions with a flick of the pen. They said they had been resolved to do the right thing, and that they had the best health advice. 'There was just no room for stress, or ego. It was just a matter of taking the information, then arriving at the best course of action,' one premier said.

For his part, Morrison offered a recent memory about life as a former prime minister. He had been watching a television show with his wife, Jenny, called *This England*. The series is a dramatisation of the first wave of Covid in the UK. It re-enacts Boris Johnson's handling of the crisis, and depicts, close up, the human impact of the failure to take swift action to slow the spreading coronavirus.

'The images from the nursing homes were … I found them quite triggering to watch,' Morrison said. 'I had to turn away. It just brought it all back.' He said that he found the period of the Victorian aged-care outbreaks in 2020, when more than 800 people died, the most difficult in the pandemic. However, he said the show also helped underline for him the success of Australia's pandemic management, compared to countries that it usually had so much in common with.

Almost 20,000 British aged-care residents died of Covid in the first few months of 2020.

'Even as bad as that was [here], what was occurring overseas was so many magnitudes above,' Morrison said. 'The actual relative international performance of the country was of little comfort at the time. Perhaps, over time, it will be a little more appreciated.'

Morrison said that he has never accepted that managing the pandemic would be a matter of choosing between economic and health priorities. 'And I think that's what Australia got right more than any other country in the world.'

Through the first two years of the pandemic, fewer people died in Australia than would usually be expected. In 2020, there was a reduction in suicides, fatal drug overdoses, and car crashes. Lockdowns, border closures, and other public health measures suppressed not just Covid, but a host of other infectious diseases that usually claimed the lives of vulnerable people. Just two deaths were recorded from the flu in Australia in 2021, for example, compared to almost 1,000 the year before the pandemic struck.

However, when Australia's death toll did start climbing again, it did so in dramatic fashion. In 2022, when many declared they were done with Covid, about 13,000 people died with or from the virus, rocketing Covid from a minor cause of death to one of Australia's biggest killers. The median age of death from Covid was just over 85 years, but also among the dead were dozens of people in their 30s or younger, and many hundreds of people in their 50s and 60s.

The effect of Covid-19 was so pronounced that it caused a temporary decline in Australia's life expectancy, knocking off about five months from the average lifespan, while recorded deaths rose about 17 per cent above the historical average. Most of these 'excess deaths' in Australia were directly caused by severe Covid, but not all of them. There were also hundreds more people than expected dying from heart disease, diabetes, and other causes. An analysis by the Actuaries Institute, which represents the profession that assesses risk for business, theorised that lingering health complications from the virus and delays in receiving emergency care might have been partly behind the increase.

While Covid-19 made fewer headlines than before, it continued to cause many hundreds of beds in Australia's hospitals to be filled, alongside a new wave of sick patients who hadn't got the care they had needed earlier in the pandemic. The nation's healthcare system, which was already running at or beyond capacity before Covid, was in crisis. Ambulances were taking longer to get to sick patients, as queues of stretchers spilled out of hospitals and into marquees in hospital car parks.

Australian Medical Association president Professor Steve Robson said that pulling together a hospital staff roster was proving almost impossible. 'One of the things that's been shocking for many health-care workers is going to work and facing these incredible pressures … their leave is cancelled, they are working double shifts … and they leave [work], and they hear political leaders and business leaders saying, "Oh, nothing to see here,"' he said. 'I think that has been a shock to a lot of healthcare workers, that perhaps there is a sense that they don't matter … and hospitals are absolutely stretched beyond the breaking point, but that's okay, it's the cost of doing business.'

In October 2022, mandatory isolation for those with Covid-19 was scrapped entirely, which meant, legally at least, that Australians were not required to stay at home and away from the public when they had the virus. Australia's chief medical officer, Professor Paul Kelly, had been asked by Australia's new prime minister, Anthony Albanese, to provide advice on the matter. Kelly said that this advice was among the most difficult he had given during the entire pandemic.

'There is no question that quarantine and isolation has been an important component of our response,' he said. 'It decreased the risk of transmission to others. In the context that we were in earlier in the pandemic, it made a lot of sense.' However, Kelly said he was getting the same feeling he had during the first summer's Omicron wave: many people were growing tired of the restrictions, and might not have been testing for Covid-19 at all. 'We've moved to a different policy intent now that's not about transmission; it's about protection of vulnerable people in high-risk settings,' he said in late 2022. He cautiously recommended to the nation's leaders the end of mandatory isolation, with the caveat that it might have to be reinstated if a new variant emerged.

The decision by the national cabinet to end forced isolation for most Australians marked a change of approach to the country's handling of the pandemic in more ways than one. The Australian Health Protection Principal Committee (AHPPC), which had been central to shaping the nation's early response to the pandemic, was sidelined. Their views were not just ignored, but not sought. A number of senior health sources told us that a meeting of the AHPPC had been scheduled the day before national cabinet was due to meet, but was cancelled.

Although his opinion wasn't officially sought, Victoria's chief health officer, Brett Sutton, sent a tweet shortly before the national cabinet decision was made public. 'Sleepwalking into Covid is not a strategy I would recommend. Still much remains uncertain,' he wrote, while sharing an article warning that new Covid-19 waves could be coming. Most interpreted this as a pointed indication of his displeasure with national cabinet's move. The Victorian government would not confirm that they had sought advice from Sutton before the decision, but in an August 2022 email to senior Victorian health department officials (obtained subsequently using freedom-of-information laws), Sutton had written, 'Omicron is substantially different to earlier variants, and isolation remains a key pillar of control.'

Sutton later told us that it had become very challenging to keep people engaged with the question of how they might reduce their risk from Covid. 'There aren't many countries that are doing extraordinary things, because there isn't a willingness in the population to do that,' he said. 'There's still a significant proportion of the community who want daily information or weekly information; we're providing that.

But there are also people who really can't hear the word [Covid] again and really don't want to engage anymore, so there's a need to kind of find a balance.' He added that he was still pushing the importance of vaccines, improving building ventilation, and encouraging people to wear a mask. These were fairly low-cost measures that had the potential to make a big difference to a pandemic that was still causing more than 100 deaths in Victoria each week, he pointed out. 'But the reality is, there's less willingness for people to disrupt their lives,' he said.

When the first national cabinet meeting of 2023 rolled around, Covid-19 wasn't on the agenda for the first time since the cabinet was founded almost three years earlier. 'I actually asked for it to be, because I thought it was appropriate that we have an update,' said ACT chief minister Andrew Barr. 'But I was unsuccessful in that regard.'

It had not been expected that Australia would snap back to life as it was before Covid. There would be a 'new normal', observers predicted. One epidemiologist had mused that children in the future would probably find it strange that in 2018 people had not worn masks when they went to the supermarket. Soldiering on and going to work with a sniffle would be seen as a 'relic of a naive society', and it was hoped that hundreds of preventable deaths from the flu in aged care would no longer be accepted as the normal course of things. It was therefore somewhat surprising to see many Australians reverting to pre-pandemic behaviour, and how high the tolerance was for deaths, including of many thousands in aged care. Those still wearing masks in the supermarket were a minority.

Dr Mark Veitch, Tasmania's director of public health, felt it had been difficult transitioning from a society that had been heavily governed by Covid-19 mandates to having virtually none at all. 'When we took away mandates for various things like masks and vaccines … what you're getting reflected back at you is, "If you're not saying I must do this, then I don't need to, and I won't."'

At the same time, there was no great attempt to drive lasting reform that could have helped save lives as Australia switched to living with Covid, such as improved building ventilation and frank messaging to Australians about the scale of the problem they were still facing. There was a disappointing lack of curiosity about the impacts of repeated waves of disease and how we might do better. Come 2023, Doherty Institute director Professor Sharon Lewin said that troubling gaps still remained in the way Australia collected information, which meant there was no clear national picture of exactly who was dying, who was suffering from long Covid, or even how many people were being infected. (The federal government was also concerned about this issue, and had vowed to take action.) 'If you look at countries like the UK, Israel, and Portugal, they have systems where they are able to analyse their data in real time,' Lewin said. 'It's an area we did very poorly in.'

There had also yet to be any concerted attempt to learn from Australia's pandemic response by investigating the impact of the various measures brought in to curtail the coronavirus. There was, for example, no thorough examination of the efficacy of controversial measures in Victoria, such as curfews, closed playgrounds, and a five-kilometre rule. Lewin reflected that it was 'extraordinary, and almost unheard of globally' that Victoria's second wave had been eradicated in 2020 with public health measures. 'But the fact is we don't know the answer to how we did it.'

So what are some of the lessons of Australia's pandemic experience? This is a complex question to answer, as we know the extraordinary steps taken to keep the virus at bay caused deep harm to some Australians, and not every place and every person was sheltered from disaster. Yet, as we have travelled across the country hearing the stories of leaders, scientists, and everyday Australians, several things have become clear.

We know with certainty that the first iteration of Covid-19 that emerged from China in early 2020 was possible to contain. This was proven in China itself, which was able to bring its outbreak under control in 2020 as the virus swept across the globe. And it was further underlined by the surprising success of Australia's national lockdown, and in Victoria the same year, when residents complied with months-long restrictions on their freedoms of movement to extinguish an outbreak that had seemed unstoppable. We will never know for sure what would have happened if Chinese authorities had acted on the counsel of scientists who told them in early January 2020 that they were dealing with another SARS-like disease, but there was a chance to stop the pandemic before it began, and it was squandered.

In Australia, almost without fail, the authorities were able to prevent devastating Covid outbreaks taking root by stopping the disease making landfall entirely, or by clamping down quickly when it did. In contrast, the long lockdowns all followed delays in taking drastic steps to stop the virus spreading. There was an interval of more than a month from when Covid leaked out of a Melbourne quarantine hotel to when the city went into a widespread lockdown in July 2020. Australia's deadly Delta outbreak of 2021 started when the New South Wales government chose to ignore the advice of its own public experts to institute a snap lockdown. Even Australia's first and only national lockdown from March 2020 could have been avoided, many experts argue, if the Australian government had listened to the epidemiologists agitating to shut the international border sooner.

From the very beginning, there were influential individuals lobbying against action, either underplaying its seriousness or baulking at the cost of the interventions. 'We can't stop living because of a flu-like virus', former Victorian premier Jeff Kennett told *The Australian* newspaper shortly before the 2020 Australian Grand Prix was cancelled. 'Yes, it might be as, or more, contagious than other flus we have been subjected to, but people can decide for themselves how they respond to any threat … Start the engines. Life does not stop for a virus or a war.' But throughout the Covid pandemic, communities and the economy inevitably paid heavier costs when governments sat on their hands and let the virus spread through an unvaccinated population.

Lockdowns and border closures were not a part of Australia's pandemic plan before 2020, but they will and should be an option in the future. That is not to say that we should shut down upon receiving every new report of a strange new coughing disease. As epidemiologist James Trauer pointed out to us, not every pandemic requires such disruptive steps. The 2009 H1N1 swine flu outbreak, which had a fatality rate of about 0.02 per cent, would be one such example. Alternatively, MERS, another type of coronavirus, has a much higher fatality rate of more than 35 per cent. Here, the case could be much stronger for swift border closures or lockdowns to suppress outbreaks while a vaccine is designed and distributed.

Trauer said the key to responding to future pandemics was assessing the threat early and making a clear choice between aiming for the elimination of the virus — the strategy that was attempted in Australia during the first years of the Covid pandemic — or mitigation to slow the spread of the disease. Covid has shown it is better to crack down fast in the face of a deadly contagion, and to risk accusations of overreach, than to wait until the situation has gotten so bad that it's too late to stop it.

Officially, almost 7 million people had died from Covid-19 worldwide at the time of this book's publication. However, the real pandemic death toll was thought to be significantly higher — possibly beyond 20 million. Many deaths were not counted in government statistics, while other people perished from other Covid-related causes, as hospitals overflowed. The majority of deaths occurred in Asia, where most of the world's population lives, but the highest death toll per capita occurred in Europe, Latin America, and North America.

Acting quickly and decisively takes courage, because it often involves taking steps before being absolutely certain they are needed. Many of the biggest pandemic decisions in Australia — to close borders and to shut down life as we knew it — were made well before the situation had spiralled into a catastrophe. As former health minister Greg Hunt pointed out, when the federal government decided to close the border to most arrivals from China in February 2020, they based their call on what the modelling was telling them might happen. At that point, there had been only about 12,000 confirmed cases of Covid-19 worldwide. 'That was an enormous leap of faith,' Hunt said.

Professor Brendan Crabb, the chief executive of the Burnet Institute, a medical research centre involved in Covid modelling, said that Scott Morrison, Greg Hunt, Gladys Berejiklian, Daniel Andrews, and the other state premiers deserved enormous credit for choosing not to follow the same path as the US and the UK early in the pandemic. Crabb said that Morrison would have had the same sort of voices in his ear as his counterparts in the US and UK, telling him that the virus was not significant enough, and that it would be possible to weather it, yet Australia still acted by closing the borders and then the country in March 2020.

'A lot of people are alive because of that. A lot less people have long Covid because of that,' he said. 'What they didn't expect was that it would actually eliminate the virus from the whole country. None of us expected that, but it worked. And so, from then on, most of the country lived virus-free until Omicron came along. [There were border closures and they were a big issue], but they were free to go to pubs, free to go to the footy, free to mix with family and friends without masks or testing, because there was no virus in most places in Australia. Of course, there were massive exceptions, but that point is often missed.'

This lesson, of prevention being better than cure, also extends to global action on addressing the factors that heighten the risk of a new virus spilling over from animals to humans in the first place, including climate change, habitat destruction, intensive agriculture, and wild-animal trading.

Illustrating just how readily predictable something like the Covid pandemic was, in 2014 Australian scientist Eddie Holmes stood at the very place that likely spawned the 2019 Covid pandemic — the south-west corner of the Wuhan Huanan Seafood Wholesale Market. Once or twice a year, Holmes would travel around China with his long-term Chinese colleague Professor Yong-Zhen Zhang, sampling viruses from many different animal species, and trying to improve our understanding of how viruses evolve and emerge in new species. One afternoon, they were driving around Wuhan looking for wetland areas when Zhang and other members of his team offered to show him what they thought was an academically interesting interaction between animals and humans.

When he got there, his attention was drawn to small side alleys trailing off into the gloom. There he found cages and cages of wild animals stacked upon each other: snakes, birds, and mammals. 'I said, "This is zoonosis waiting to happen. They're basically pooing on each other, and the viruses are going to spread,"' Holmes remembered.

In other words, he came close to predicting the pandemic, probably at its very source.

The virologist was particularly bothered by the presence of raccoon dogs. These fluffy and intelligent creatures with dark eyes are bred for their fur, and have been linked to SARS. 'I knew they shouldn't be in the market,' he said. With his iPhone, he furtively took a photo of three of the animals huddled in the back of a cage, their eyes red from the flash of the camera, sitting above a cage of birds he couldn't identify.

That same year, one of the authors of this book penned an article for *The Age* newspaper in Melbourne. Based on government pandemic-planning documents and expert interviews, it began like this: 'A deadly pandemic could shut down Melbourne as we know it. Public transport could be terminated, AFL games cancelled and the casino, schools and office towers forced to close.' This was in 2014, more than five years before the Covid pandemic began.

The article forecast that mass vaccination centres would be set up across the city, and warned that funeral directors might have to videotape services so friends of the deceased could watch at home as part of a policy of 'social distancing' (a phrase so unfamiliar at the time that it was put in quotation marks). Predictably, this article has been held up by conspiracy theorists as evidence that the pandemic was deliberately started by humans—a 'plan-demic'. But we know that most of the destructive future events that will harm Australia and the world are entirely foreseeable. If we don't listen to scientists when they urge us and our governments to change our behaviour, many more of these dystopian headlines will come to life.

Holmes said one of the reforms that should come out of the 2019 pandemic was the establishment of a global surveillance system that would allow people to upload the information they had about possible emerging diseases in real time. 'The clear lesson out of the Covid-19 debacle is that scientists and governments should feel empowered to share data as quickly as possible', he said. 'If they had done that in Wuhan earlier, they might have clamped down earlier, and we might have never got the pandemic.' However, as the debate over the origins of the Covid-19 pandemic became intensely politicised, confused, and clouded by xenophobia, racism, and blame, Holmes said his colleagues in China were much less able to speak freely. Because of this, the swift sharing of information is more out of reach than it was before. 'We are ten times more unsafe now,' he said.

In 1918, Australia was able to withstand the Spanish Flu pandemic better than much of the rest of the world, by virtue of its isolation and its maritime quarantine program. Troop ships carrying returning World War I soldiers and other vessels arriving from infected countries had to quarantine for seven days, and passengers were subject to 'daily thermometer parades'. But come 2020, the world had changed, and policy-makers could have been forgiven for thinking that the lessons of this old crisis would not apply to a globalised world in which countries were connected by a single plane flight rather than a lengthy sea voyage. Yet, as infectious disease expert Professor Allen Cheng said, it was a mistake not to retain purpose-built

accommodation for 21st-century pandemics. 'We didn't have quarantine facilities, because we didn't think we would need them, and it
wasn't really seen as an option,' Cheng said.

As it turned out, Australia's position, sea-locked and near the
bottom of the world, meant it remained uniquely placed to fend off
a pandemic. But the absence of dedicated quarantine facilities left
state governments relying mostly on cramped hotels with shared
hallways to house the infected travellers, leading to regular virus
escapes that constantly threatened Australia's pre-vaccine pandemic
strategy. By the time new dedicated facilities were built in Victoria,
Queensland, and Western Australia, the need for mass quarantining
of travellers had already passed.

Once, Australia had many quarantine facilities: for example, a
station at Victoria's Port Nepean with a morgue and wooden huts
for influenza patients harboured the victims of typhus and scarlet
fever in the 1850s, and became a temporary home for hundreds of
refugees from the Bosnian War in the 1990s; and, over 100 years
ago, thousands of returning World War I soldiers were sent to Bruny
Island off the coast of Tasmania for fumigation. But, by 2020, the
many outposts once dedicated to infectious disease quarantine had
become historical artefacts. Ghost tours were held at the old North
Head Quarantine Station in Manly in New South Wales, since
refashioned into a hotel.

There is also something else worth remembering about Australia's
make-up, which is difficult to capture in any official plans and
reports: the psyche of its people, which was so central to the country's success in dealing with the first phase of the pandemic.

'Australians don't mind rules and regulations. Some people talk
about it being a nanny state,' explained pandemic adviser Professor
James McCaw. 'We're not allowed to install our own electricity
wires, but in the UK of course you can do your home wiring. There's
all sorts of things that people who come from outside Australia are
surprised by that we take for granted. But I actually think they're
part of a culture that means that we respond very well to things

like pandemics. We trust governments, and we want to do the right thing.'

At its worst, this penchant for rule-following manifested itself in police fining thousands of people for rule minor infractions, and in citizens dobbing on their neighbours. But, at its best, it achieved what had seemed impossible: avoiding tens of thousands of deaths because Australians were willing to make enormous sacrifices for the collective good. Western Australian premier Mark McGowan put this another way. He said Australians as a people 'have a very low tolerance for mistakes, or for people dying when it was avoidable. In this country, perhaps more than any other place in the world, we value people's lives.'

At the start of the pandemic, there had been a flippant refrain that while our grandparents went to war to protect their country, all this generation needed to do was sit at home on the couch for a few weeks. What eventuated was not a fleeting crisis, but a vast, expanding disaster producing chronic stress, disruption, and losses over several years. Still, sometimes the nation's response to the Covid crisis was tunnel-visioned. Not enough effort was put into helping people cope mentally. Too often, rules were enforced in a way that seemed unnecessarily cruel, most notably when people were prevented from being with their dying loved ones during their final moments.

Australia might be colloquially known as the 'lucky country', but not everyone felt the effects of the coronavirus pandemic equally. Lower socio-economic communities, the culturally and linguistically diverse, and those with insecure but essential work were infected, hospitalised, impoverished, and killed at far higher rates by Covid. This was laid out starkly at times in 2021, when intensive-care units at some of Melbourne and Sydney's major hospitals were filled exclusively with patients from Middle Eastern backgrounds. Entire families were in hospital beds scattered across wards, and hooked up to ventilators.

Along the way, governments often failed to communicate with Australians from migrant backgrounds in their own language and through the right avenues, such as trusted community leaders. This was particularly pronounced during the vaccine rollout, leaving a vacuum for misinformation to spread. Entrenched inequality also meant that it was harder for migrants to protect themselves in the first place. The backbone of the nation's insecure and casualised workforce, they were unable to retreat to their home offices, and were exposed to the virus at the highest rate of the entire population.

Psychiatrist Professor Patrick McGorry said that in any major infectious-disease outbreak in the future, the needs of young people and children, and the mental health of the entire population, had to be at the forefront of any response. In future disasters, he hoped to see a chief psychiatrist by the side of every chief health officer. 'In other words, we've got to think about all aspects of the health of the whole population,' McGorry said. 'We've got to think more about the non-fatal impacts on the community. That is suffering and disability, blighted lives and futures, not just pure mortality.'

Epidemiologist James Trauer said it should have been the case that children were the last to be impacted by public health interventions, 'whereas they often bore the brunt of the restrictions. This isn't to say that school closures were never appropriate — they were probably needed to achieve elimination in Victoria in 2020. But for Covid, school closures should have consistently been the last restriction implemented, and the first one released.'

Another issue that will almost certainly be examined in future inquiries is the role of state border closures, which were undoubtedly the key to shielding the country's smaller states from disasters. Federal health minister Mark Butler told us he remained struck by the 'very weird' period in the second half of 2021, when he felt there were essentially two Australias. One was made up of the majority of Australia's population, in Sydney, Melbourne, and Canberra, stuck in extended lockdowns and exposed to the virus. The other was made up of the remaining states and territories, including his home state of South Australia. From the state's capital, Adelaide, he was able to travel freely to all the other zero-Covid states: Queensland, Western Australia, Tasmania, and the Northern Territory.

'In Western Australia, they were all in the footy stadium, with no masks, drinking beer, having a hoot of a time,' Butler said. 'I'll tell you what, the people of WA will say, "Close the border, just close it." It worked for those states, and worked for those governments. There's no question in my mind, all of those governments will be saying, "We will do it again, in a heartbeat."'

However, a key lesson of the Covid border closures is the clear need for nuance and humanity in our responses to future crises. We must strive to never have a situation again where gravely ill Australians are delayed from seeking urgent medical care at hospitals across the border, or where children are separated from their parents. Contingency plans assisting people to be with their dying loved ones should be at the heart of any response.

This book has detailed an extraordinary time in our country's history. There were great tragedies and avoidable deaths. Many Australians said goodbye to life as they knew it, and faced a reality that seemed more akin to science fiction. They had to deal with rules that were so severe that people could no longer work, or go to school, or travel outside their neighbourhood; the sound of postcodes being read out by their premier, sending thousands back into lockdown; hotels stacked high with returned travellers, holed up in rooms for two weeks at a time; and rows of patients lying face-down in intensive care, who feared the vaccine more than the virus.

But the reality is that many of the terrible stories that we might have told about the coronavirus pandemic in Australia will never need to be written. An analysis by epidemiologist James Trauer found that up to 60,000 lives were probably saved because Australia adopted an elimination strategy before vaccinations became available. He came to this figure using the death rates in Europe and North America, where, by 2023, 1,500 to 3,200 people in every million had died of Covid. If Australia had responded similarly to these countries, he said, we would have seen in the order of 40,000 to 80,000 Covid deaths, rather than about 20,000, in the pandemic's first three years.

He said it was also very important to note that those countries in Europe and North America did try to keep the virus at bay to varying degrees, even though they weren't as successful as Australia. For example, Britain had three national lockdowns, with strict rules in place for about six months. Trauer said that the results of a genuine 'do-nothing' approach in Australia were harder to guesstimate, but he said that, based on an infection rate of 80 per cent, he would have expected between 100,000 to 250,000 deaths, not including those who died from other causes because there were no beds available at overrun hospitals.

So what exactly would an uncontrolled Covid-19 catastrophe have looked like in Australia? What stories would we be telling now if, back in March 2020, the nation had continued on the same path it was on—just a little behind Britain, France, Germany, and the United States? We can try to imagine this by looking at these countries and transposing their stories, or by taking Australia's coronavirus disasters and multiplying them. But this probably wouldn't create the right picture. A likely scenario would have seen the impacts of Australia's coronavirus crisis inverted, with least populated states worst impacted, instead of faring the best.

The Northern Territory, with its small population, tiny health care system, and many poorly serviced Aboriginal communities, would have been overwhelmed quickly. The director of epidemiology at the Doherty Institute, Professor Jodie McVernon, said little had been published in the US about the impact of Covid on its First Nations peoples, but what there was 'wasn't good'. McVernon theorised that Australia's hospitals would have been able to retain higher care standards for a little longer than in the UK, where the National Health Service had been decimated by years of funding cutbacks. Outbreaks may have been somewhat constrained in the warmer parts of the nation, because Covid in the tropics never seemed to take off like it did in the south-eastern states. But, as happened worldwide, the harm from the pandemic would have fallen even more savagely on marginalised and disadvantaged Australians, on migrants and front-line workers, while wealthier Australians bunkered down at home.

'We would have seen a lot of deaths,' McVernon said. 'There was nothing special or magical about us.' The epidemiologist said perhaps the time has come to reflect positively on the harms that were averted in Australia. She had been in meetings in early 2020 with many of the other leading disease-modellers around the world, and all of them were giving the same advice to their governments. 'Australia benefited from the fact that our politicians listened,' she said. 'And I think social cohesion in Australia was remarkable. People did, on the whole, cooperate, and they did think communally, collectively, even though it was really, really tough.'

Acknowledgements

We are so grateful to so many for helping and encouraging us to write this book.

We will forever appreciate the love and support of our families, who perhaps didn't realise what they were in for when we optimistically declared that we would be taking 'a couple of months off work' to write a book.

This book wouldn't have been possible without Aisha's husband, Charles Gaylard, who offered his unwavering support, taking on the role of chief parent for many months as the book consumed countless weekends, nights, and holidays. Thank you, too, to Max and Henry Gaylard, for their patience and for providing joyful entertainment during our long workdays.

A massive thank you goes to our chief sub-editor, Aisha's dad, Dr Alastair Dow, who was the first person to read our manuscript, in its many versions, over almost a year. Alastair, you have helped us more than you'll ever know with your encyclopaedic knowledge and sharp and considered edits. It was really special having you as part of the process.

Melissa would like to thank her mum, Jan, who has always believed; her wisdom, kindness, and mighty heart have always guided Melissa in everything she does. And she would also like to thank her dad, Chris, for his unwavering love and support; he has instilled in her an unquenchable curiosity for life, and taught her that every story always begins and ends with people. Thanks to Bec, for her endless support and being the best sister, and to Josh and Adam, for all their love and encouragement. Melissa would also like to thank many of her friends who have always been there for her, but especially in the last year, offering support, love, and laughs. Special mention to Molly Perrett and Laura Alston for their never-ending support and countless check-ins in the past 12 months during the challenges of writing the book.

Aisha would like to thank her mother, Rose, who provided both moral and practical support for this project, and who has always lovingly encouraged and been engaged in her children's careers and interests. The same can be said for her parents-in-law, Elizabeth and Geoffrey, who have been great supporters and help. Thank you, too, to Aisha's brother, Angus, her sisters-in-law, brothers-in-law, and her friends for their interest and ideas.

We are so grateful for the support of our colleagues at *The Age*, who generously put us in touch with their contacts, allowed us to take many months off work during a busy news period, and offered their counsel on everything from the book's title to publishing contacts. We also drew on their extensive and brilliant reporting of the pandemic for our book. A huge thank you goes to Kate Lahey, who was instantly enthusiastic about this project, even though it meant being a staff member short. Kate read and edited many chapters of the book, and her amazing support, and intelligent and thoughtful insights, have been invaluable. We would also like to thank Ben Schneiders, Konrad Marshall, Deb Cuthbertson, Patrick Elligett, Henrietta Cook, Melissa Singer, Simone Fox Koob, Marija Ercegovac, Miki Perkins, Liam Mannix, James Massola, Kate Aubusson, Rachael Dexter, Gay Alcorn, Sumeyya Ilanbey, Caroline Hartnett, Michael Lynch, and Chip Le Grand.

There are too many others to name, but dozens of people across *The Age* and *Sydney Morning Herald* newsrooms helped us in ways big and small. We also received generous help from journalists in other newsrooms, particularly Andrew Hough, who answered many fact-checking questions.

This book wouldn't have been possible without the time and generosity of the many people who agreed to be interviewed for this book, from scientists to healthcare workers, politicians, and ordinary Australians who had extraordinary stories to share. We will be forever grateful to them. We are indebted to the family members of those who lost their loved ones during the pandemic and who bravely shared their stories with us.

Finally, our immense gratitude goes to our publisher, Henry Rosenbloom, who backed our pitch from the very beginning and took a chance on two first-time authors. Henry's patience, expert guidance, and thoughtful edits were instrumental in bringing this monumental project to life.

Index